Sirt Diet

Your All-Purpose Guide to a Balanced Sirt Diet, Including the Science Behind the Approach, Step-By-Step Walkthroughs, Recipes, and more!

MAX CALIGARI

TABLE OF CONTENTS

Introduction 1

Chapter 1: The Possibilities of the Sirt Diet, and Why Everyone is Talking About It.. 3

Chapter 2: The Science Behind the Sirt Diet.............. 16

Chapter 3: The Potential Health and Weight Loss Benefits 28

Chapter 4: Empowering Yourself with Sirt Foods 45

Chapter 5: Succeeding with Phase One..................... 75

Chapter 6: Reaching Your Goals with Phase Two 86

Chapter 7: How to Continue Managing Your Weight and Promoting the Sirt Lifestyle 91

Chapter 8: Questions and Answers for Success......... 94

Chapter 9: Simple and Delicious Recipes to Get You Started... 99

Conclusion 120

INTRODUCTION

The Sirt diet is full of superfoods in a class known as 'sirtfoods.' While scientists have known for a long time that these foods have healing and weight loss proprieties, they have only been put together into a single diet in recent years. A handful if sirtfoods include:

- Dark chocolate
- Red wine
- Green tea
- Blueberries
- Turmeric
- Kale
- Parsley
- And more

The creators of the Sirt diet, two dietitians from the UK, formed these specific coined the term 'sirtfood' and combined it into a single diet specifically to target weight loss. This was done after research found that sirtfoods are high in sirtuins, a type of protein found not only within certain foods but also in the human body. These proteins have a powerful effect on weight loss, metabolism, inflammation, and the body's natural aging process. The result is that you can lose more weight while retaining muscle and health.

You may have recently heard about the Sirt diet after Adele's fantastic transformation. While the diet had previously helped many people, it was still relatively unheard of by most individuals until Adele attributed her success to the plan. The standard plan following the Sirt diet consists of two phases lasting a length of a week each. This can help people lose weight quickly when needed, such as if they are trying to get their high cholesterol or blood pressure down before a date set by their doctor or lose a certain number of pounds to their dream wedding dress or tux. However, there is another method of the Sirt diet. You can also follow for slower and more sustained weight loss. This version is ideal for people who able to take a little more time for weight loss that is just as effective yet more sustainable. Whichever version of the Sirt diet you plan to choose, the traditional or the innovative (or a combination of both!), I will provide you with a step-by-step guide to gently walk you through the process. You can attain the success you desire, whether you want to lose weight or boost your health.

CHAPTER 1: THE POSSIBILITIES OF THE SIRT DIET, AND WHY EVERYONE IS TALKING ABOUT IT

The Sirt diet first made the news when Pipa Middleton used it, combined with daily palates, to lose weight before her wedding. However, it really took the world by storm more recently, when Adele attributed her successful fifty-pound loss to the plan. However, while people may have gained a little understanding of what the diet partially entails, most are still largely in the dark. But don't worry! I will provide you with everything you need to know to attain success with the Sirt diet, whether you choose to attempt the fast-paced traditional approach or the tailored long-term sustainable approach. Both the traditional and my method have pros and cons. But, by having the information regarding each method, you can choose the option that is best for your individual circumstances. We will begin by exploring the very basics of the Sirt food diet. I will provide you with Sirt Diet 101. By having this knowledge, you will then be able to dive deeper into the later chapters.

When you begin the Sirt diet, you will start to lose weight quickly due to eating nutrient-rich foods, a reduced calorie intake, and, of course, select ingredients high in the sirtuin proteins. This innovative approach is known to activate a person's "skinny gene," which are natural pathways in the human body that are typically only activated by exercise and fasting. Foods that are high in the sirtuins, a form of natural polyphenols found within the human body and certain foods, mimic the effect of fasting and exercise by pushing our cells to burn more fat. Whether you are eating dark chocolate, kale, turmeric, or red wine (in moderation), you can push your cells to burn more fat while maintaining valuable lean muscle tone and improving overall health. Not only will your metabolism be revved into gear, but these Sirtfoods have also been found to promote healthy aging and positive moods.

Once you attain your goal weight, you can effectively maintain a sustained goal weight by eating your recommended caloric intake for your body mass index and activity level, along with continuing to include Sirtfoods in your diet. By eating a standard balanced diet with nutritious foods, and including Sirtfoods, you will be able to maintain the weight loss you achieved even when you enjoy the occasional "cheat day" or a less than nutritionally recommended meal. This doesn't mean you should eat as many calories or as much junk food as you want, as long as you also eat Sirtfoods, but it does give you more flexibility and freedom to maintain your goal weight while also enjoying life and food to the fullest.

When you begin the Sirtfood diet, you will follow two simple step-by-step phases. During the first phase, which traditionally lasts seven days, you will start by consuming very few calories. The first three days of the first phase will provide you with three servings of sirtuin-rich green juice and a single large meal daily. This results in a total of one-thousand calories each of the first three days. During the fourth, through the seventh day of the first phase, you will increase your caloric intake. You will now consume two meals and two green juices for a total of fifteen-hundred calories. It is during the first phase that you will lose the most weight.

It is important to note that while red wine is high in sirtuins, you will not be consuming any alcohol during the first phase of the Sirt diet, as alcohol can also hinder weight loss. For this reason, red wine is only for the second phase. Although, in the first phase, you can still enjoy plenty of water, green juice, green tea, and coffee.

The second phase of the Sirt diet is designed for weight maintenance. You will consume; however, many calories are recommended for your BMI (body-mass index) and activity level. These calories will be in the form of one daily green juice and three healthy/balanced meals. While you have a great amount of freedom as to what these meals consist of, you should try to include plenty of fruits, vegetables, and of course, Sirtfoods.

If you are looking to lose a lot of weight, then with the traditional Sirt diet method, you will first follow the first phase, followed by fourteen days in the second phase. After the second phase, you will repeat the first and second phase again, as following this pattern as many times as needed until you reach your goal weight. You shouldn't follow the first phase longer than recommended, as it is really low in calories, and by combining it with the second phase, you can ensure you consume the nutrients your body requires to thrive.

You can follow the second phase for the standard fourteen days or indefinitely. If you choose to follow this phase for a set amount of time and then wish to maintain your weight loss, you can Sirtify your diet. To do this, you consume a standard calorie intake and healthy balanced meals, but you include elements of the Sirt diet, as well. For instance, while you can now eat three meals a day, you should still drink your daily Sirt-rich green juice. Along with the juice, you should also look for ways to add more Sirt foods to your daily meals. Whether you are eating a salad, pancakes, pasta, pitta, or burritos, look for ways you can add in a couple of servings of Sirt ingredients each meal to continue maintaining your weight and health. You will find that doing this increases the flavor of your meals, as foods full of sirtuins are also full of flavor. Later on, I will provide you with a number of recipes full of sirtuins that you can enjoy.

One key aspect of the Sirt diet is the green juice you will be drinking daily. This is important, as it provides you with a large number of Sirtfoods in a single glass. You absolutely can not skip the green juice. Thankfully, it is simple to make! I recommend starting out your morning, making all the green juice you will drink for the day, which you can then store in the fridge. This will save you time and energy so that you don't have to use and clean your juicer three times a day, but it will still maximize the nutrients in the juice by keeping it fresh. You don't want to make juice any more than a day in advance, as if you store it for longer than twenty-four hours, the nutrients will begin to breakdown, making the juice less effective.

You can't use a juicer for the green juice, as it will not prepare it correctly. However, you can find good deals on juicers online if you look. Along with a juicer, you will also need a digital kitchen scale, as the juice is prepared with weight measurements. Weight-based measuring is important, as it is much more accurate, especially for ingredients such as kale and arugula.

The ingredients for green juice are usually pretty simple to find in a nearby store or online. You find arugula (rocket variety), kale, parsley, celery, green apples, ginger root, and lemons in nearly any produce department. You will also need matcha green tea (different from regular green tea), which you can either find on the tea aisle of a grocery store, but it is also readily available online. Lastly, it is ideal if you can add in the herb lovage. However, this herb is not easy to find in American stores, so if you choose to use it for the best results, then you will need to buy seeds online. Thankfully, lovage can easily be grown in small pots in a yard, on a balcony, or even on your kitchen windowsill.

If you're like me, you are most likely wondering about now what your actual meals will look like. After all, the drink options might be nice and all, but there is just no beating a good meal. The good news is that the

Sirt diet is full of not only ingredients rich in sirtuins, but you can eat other healthy and nutritious ingredients, as well. For instance, if you have some whole grains and salmon on hand, you can enjoy them with a peach ginger compote and a massaged kale salad topped with lemon juice, olive oil, ginger, blueberries, parsley, walnuts, and celery. This meal is not only really well balanced and universally accepted as healthy, but it is also full of a number of Sirtfoods. It's important to remember that the list of Sirtfoods (which we will get to shortly) are not the only foods you are allowed to eat. You can enjoy other healthy whole foods as well; you simply need to prioritize eating a large number of Sirt-rich ingredients to promote optimal weight loss.

Some optional meal ideas include:
- Soy yogurt topped with dark chocolate, toasted walnuts, and fresh berries
- Omelet filled with parsley, kale, radicchio, and chilies
- Buckwheat berry pancakes
- Massaged kale salad with celery, parsley, green apple, toasted walnuts, and a vinaigrette made with lemon juice, olive oil, and fresh ginger root. Top it off with some chicken, turkey, or salmon for protein, and try adding some cooked buckwheat berries on top for a more filling meal.
- Whole-grain pitta bread stuffed with hummus, parsley, turkey, and cheese
- Buckwheat noodles tossed with kale, olive oil, walnuts, capers, and shrimp
- Lamb tagine with butternut squash and dates, served over cooked whole grains

When it comes to Sirtfood-rich meals, there are many options. They will help you lose weight while you enjoy flavorful, rich, and delicious food on a daily basis.

Now that you have an idea as to what you can expect from the Sirt diet, let's delve in a bit deeper into what Sirtfoods are and how they affect your body. As we previously mentioned, sirtuins are a type of protein naturally found within both the human body and certain foods. When you eat foods rich in sirtuins, also known as polyphenols, is causes the sirtuin gene within your body to activate, thus pushing weight loss into gear, optimizing the aging process, and providing other health benefits. Just as fasting and exercise have long been shown to increase overall health, memory, metabolism, muscle development, and blood sugar levels, so too do sirtuin-rich foods.

When you read over the list of sirtfoods, you may notice that they are all plant-based, not animal-based. This is because plants are generally stationary, causing them to develop a sophisticated system of stress-response to adapt and thrive in their natural environments. This stress-response system causes an increased number of polyphenols (sirtuins.) As it has long been said, "you are what you eat." The end result is that when you consume plants rich in sirtuins, you thereby consume the polyphenols and are able to benefit from their profound effects. Just as the polyphenols affect a plant's stress-response pathways, they will do the same in humans, as well.

However, while all plants have a stress-response system, not all plants have adapted and developed to the degree that results in a high number of sirtuins. You can't simply eat a plant-based diet and expect to consume a large number of sirtuins; you need to know which plants contain them and prioritize the consumption of those. The good news is that we now know which plants are highest in polyphenols, allowing us to not haphazardly guessing which plants may be the best choice. By understanding this knowledge, we can truly revolutionize weight loss without requiring arduous exercise programs and gym memberships or strict fasting schedules.

In many ways, sirtfoods are a new class of superfoods, which are specific ingredients that have been found to be especially dense and powerful in certain nutritional aspects. In fact, many of the ingredients on the sirtfood list have long been known to have beneficial properties for health and weight loss. For instance, you will see that ginger is frequently used in Chinese medicine, and red wine is drunk regularly in the Mediterranean, where people have been found to live longer, healthier lives. Because of this, while the Sirt diet has not been around long enough to have studies specifically targeting it, there are many studies that have been done over the decades examining the health and weight loss benefits of certain Sirt-rich foods.

Studies have found that the regular consumption of green tea can lower blood pressure, treat diabetes, and reduce the risk of stroke. Dark chocolate has been proven to reduce inflammation and lower the risk of heart disease. Turmeric is frequently used to treat chronic diseases, as studies have found it to reduce inflammation, manage autoimmune diseases, and provide general health and wellness benefits. As you can see, despite not having finished studies specifically studying the Sirt diet, we can still understand the health and weight loss benefits by finding scientific evidence relating to aspects of the plan.

Frank Hu, a professor and expert on nutrition and epidemiology at Harvard, once explained, "Substantial observational evidence exists for the beneficial effects of the intake of food and drinks rich in sirtuin activators in decreasing risks of chronic disease." The reason for this is multi-faceted. Sirtfoods have been found to promote both overall health and reduced aging of the cells. Because of this, naturally, a person who consumes a sirtuin-rich diet is less likely to develop either chronic illnesses or age-related diseases.

While sirtuins are naturally found in plants, not any plant-based ingredients will sufficiently increase your sirtuin intake. This is because only specific plants have developed to be high in this type of protein. Some fruits and vegetables you will find in the produce department, such as cucumbers, lettuce, carrots, tomatoes, avocados, kiwis, and bananas, for instance, are all incredibly low in sirtuin levels. Of course, you should still consume these fruits and vegetables, as they have other nutritional benefits and are important for a balanced diet. But, you need to understand that you have to look elsewhere if you hope to benefit from sirtuins. We will go more in-depth into the science in chapter two, so, for now, let's look at the top twenty-one foods on the Sirt diet.

Top Sirtuin-Rich Foods Include:
- Buckwheat
- Dark Chocolate/Cocoa
- Coffee
- Medjool Dates
- Kale
- Rocket Arugula
- Capers
- Extra Virgin Olive Oil

- Parsley
- Matcha Green Tea
- Celery
- Bird's Eye Chilies
- Lovage
- Radicchio
- Soy
- Turmeric
- Walnuts
- Blueberries
- Onion
- Strawberries
- Red Wine
- Black Currant
- Cherries
- Wheat Bran
- Cranberries
- Peanuts
- Rose Hips
- Dark Plums
- Red Cabbage
- Eggplant
- Cinnamon

Sirt Diet Safety and Potential Side Effects

Before ending this chapter, most of you are probably curious about the safety and potential side effects of the Sirt diet, as you should be. To put it simply, the safety and whether or not you experience side effects all depend on your personal health and what day-to-day choices you may, just like it does on any diet. The Sirt diet is usually safe. However, there are some cautions you should keep in mind in order to have the best experience possible.

Foods rich in sirtuins are also incredibly helpful superfoods that anyone could benefit from eating more of. They are high in anti-inflammatory properties and antioxidants, both of which can reduce the risk of disease and slow down cellular aging. But, if you only choose to eat foods on the Sirt food list that I provided you above, then you will not be eating a balanced diet. This is why the recipes in this book also include other fruits, vegetables, grains, and protein sources. You can not live off of only a handful of ingredients, at least not healthfully. If you try to eat only sirtuin-rich foods, you may lose more health in the short-term, but you will only experience negative long-term side effects. This is why I, again and again, promote the importance of eating a balanced Sirtfood diet.

The first phase of the Sirt diet can be restrictive, as you are eating one thousand to fifteen hundred calories a day. However, for this reason, the first phase only lasts a week and is healthy to do in the short-term. You wouldn't want to live an entire month eating that number of calories a day, but, for a week most, it is sufficient for most people. Regularly consult your family doctor before making big life changes that affect your health. Depending on your specific health, weight, and activity level, you might need to make an adjustment to a diet plan to make it work for your individual needs. Your doctor is the one most qualified to determine if you need to make these given adjustments. For instance, if you work a manual labor job, your doctor might recommend you increase your calorie and protein intake to keep your energy levels up. Remember, if your doctor does have concerns due to your individual health, it doesn't mean you can't follow the Sirt diet, simply that you need to make their recommended adjustments to your plan.

Thankfully, the average healthy adult is unlikely to have any problems with the Sirt diet if they follow it in a balanced manner recommended. This means you shouldn't increase the duration of phase one to promote further weight loss. Remember, if you want to lose more weight, then only repeat phase one after completing phase two.

For a healthy adult, the most common side effects are fatigue, irritability, and lightheadedness. This is usually due to calorie restriction and can occur whenever a person goes on a diet or changes their eating habits.

You should also know that this diet is not recommended for anyone with an eating disorder. This is because while the calorie restriction is healthy when followed according to plan, for a person who already has disordered eating, it only reinforces their negative relationship with food. The result could be that if someone with an eating disorder attempts to follow this or any other diet calling for counting calories that their eating disorder will likely worsen. Of course, if you or someone you know has an eating disorder and still wants to benefit from Sirtuin-rich foods, you can still enjoy the recipes in this book and incorporate the top Sirtfoods into your daily meal plan without cutting your calorie intake. You may not experience as much weight loss, but you have to prioritize your mental health and healing from disordered eating.

To sum it up, you should speak with your doctor before drastically changing your eating habits no matter what diet you are trying, and that includes the Sirt diet. However, if you are healthy and not pregnant, breastfeeding, or suffering from an eating disorder, it should be safe if you follow the diet as recommended. Even if you have a chronic illness or disease, it may be healthy, but only your doctor can say for sure, as each person's disease, condition, and treatment will vary.

CHAPTER 2: THE SCIENCE BEHIND THE SIRT DIET

There are multiple types and classes of sirtuins that are referred to on the Sirt diet. The first class is generally simply referred to as "sirtuins," which are those found within the human body. However, when sirtuins are found in plants, which are then consumed and can be used by people, they are known as "polyphenols." These polyphenols are organic and bioactive compounds that, while a little different from the sirtuins naturally found within humans, still result in the same biochemical process that results in increased weight loss and promote a variety of health improvements. We will now explore how sirtuins and polyphenols affect the human body and what science has proven about its benefits.

Cellular homeostasis is incredibly important for every aspect of human health. When your cells are in a state of homeostasis, it means that they are working as they should be. They are comfortable, healthy, and doing their job appropriately. They are neither underworking or overworking; everything is as it should be. When you are in cellular homeostasis, you naturally reduce excessive aging or illnesses, instead of promoting whole-body healing and wellness. A 2016 research study by Polish experts on biology, biochemistry, and plant physiology found that sirtuins play a key role in the process of cellular homeostasis, and it shouldn't be underestimated.

Let's go over some of the details of this pioneering study. Don't worry; I will skip the scientific gibberish and speak in layman's terms. Both humans and plants have cellular enzymes that act as a sensor to detect and promote homeostasis. There are different classes of these enzymes, and the third type has been dubbed "sirtuins." Not only are there two different classes of sirtuins, as we previously mentioned, there are also seven different types. These types are known simply as Sirt[number 1-7]. Each of these types has one of three roles so that they can all work together throughout the entire body.

One of the roles of some of the sirtuins is to affect the mitochondrial system. This is important, as the mitochondrial system affects a person's weight loss, healing ability, energy levels, and more. Mitochondria are known as a powerhouse. The mitochondrial systems are one of the most important aspects of maintaining homeostasis, as, without it, no human would be able to survive. Those who live with mitochondrial dysfunctions experience severe and widespread symptoms that interfere with daily life. Thankfully, this study found that sirtuins can promote a healthy mitochondrial system leading to cellular homeostasis. In particular, this can help a person increase metabolism and weight loss, reduce inflammation levels, lessen oxidative stress and cellular damage that lead to disease, and promote cellular longevity as you age. As you can imagine, by using sirtuins to activate the mitochondrial system, you not only can help manage and possibly treat mitochondrial disorders, but also other conditions such as obesity, type II diabetes, neurodegenerative diseases, cancer, and more. In part, this positive change is due to the way sirtuins are able to stimulate the mitochondria and mitochondrial proteins to prevent negative changes before they can even occur and treat them directly at the source.

Polyphenols come in a number of classifications with resveratrol and quercetin, being two of them that are more widely known. Each type can have different positive effects, meaning you want to consume sirtuins from a variety of plant-based foods to experience all of the benefits. For instance, you might have heard about resveratrol being found in grape skins and therefore wine, this resveratrol is the very same sirtuins you will be consuming on the Sirt diet. This type of sirtuin specifically has been found to positively affect the Sirt1 category within the body, leading to weight loss, reduced insulin resistance, and improved motor function.
When studying polyphenols, the researchers tracked the number of polyphenols in a given serving for plant matter and their class. For instance, the classes of polyphenols tested include flavonols, flavones, isoflavones, and more. While the researchers in this specific study were unable to test all of the high-

sirtuin foods that we mentioned in chapter one, the ones they did test reinforced what had already been proven: these foods are some of the highest in sirtuin and therefore perfect for the Sirt diet. Some other foods that the researchers proved her high in sirtuins and therefore helpful to consume more of include orange, lemon, grapefruit, eggplant, beans, blackberries, black currants, black grapes, cherries, and rhubarb.

It was also found that other foods and polyphenols can affect each other and how effectively your body absorbs and utilizes them. For instance, if you consume protein (such as meat) and polyphenols together, your body will be unable to absorb either the protein or the polyphenols, as well as it usually would. For this reason, it is a good idea to drink your green juice separately from your meals. It is still beneficial to add as many Sirtfoods to your meals as possible, even when you are eating protein, but just know that your body will not absorb as many of the sirtuins as it otherwise would. But, if you drink your green juice a couple of hours prior or after you consume protein, you will be able to ensure you get the most benefit out of it possible.

Similarly, the study also found that by heating plants through boiling, steaming, roasting, or cooking in any other way, the sirtuins and their benefits are reduced. Again, this doesn't mean you can't ever cook sirtuin-rich food, but should stay mindful of this and try to eat as many of them raw as possible.

The study concluded that sirtuins are incredibly powerful for general health and wellness, but people should keep in mind how what you consume them with and how you prepare them will affect the sirtuin levels within the food.

When you reduce caloric intake, it results in your metabolic and autophagy processes increasing. However, calorie reduction is not the only way you can experience this benefit, as a study published in Cell Death and Disease in 2010 found. This study found that when you activate your body's natural sirtuins through ingesting polyphenols, you can make use of these same important biological processes, which the researchers could be used to treat cancer in the future. Now, imagine, what if you combine caloric restriction along with increased polyphenol intake? It is likely that by combining these two aspects, both key aspects of the Sirt diet, you could compound the effects for even better results.

By restricting your calories and increasing your Sirt food intake, you can slow down the rate of cellular aging, thereby increasing not only the lifespan of your cells but possibly increase your own life span, as well. Not only that, but as it promotes overall health and wellness, and not simply living to an older age, you might be able to enjoy your golden years happier and healthier, living them to the fullest. Of course, no scientist or doctor, will guarantee you this, and neither will I, as anyone who makes such claims is only making false promises. Yet, I can promise you that science is on the side of Sirtuins and balanced calorie restriction. Study after study has found that both of these elements of the Sirt diet can increase a person's overall health and expected lifespan.

Many people have never heard of the autophagy process, despite its importance. It is a natural biochemical process of the body. Throughout human history, people have unknowingly made use of the autophagy process to help treat disease. They did this largely through fasting. Thankfully, in recent years researchers have learned more about autophagy, not only about its importance but also how we can better make use of it. No longer do we have to fast whenever we want to use this natural reaction, we can use other methods, such as calorie restriction paired with Sirt food intake, to induce it, as well.

The word "autophagy is derived from Latin, with two words combining to literally translate to "self-eating." At first appearance, it may sound like a bad idea to have your body eat itself, but I promise you, in this case, it is something you want to happen. It doesn't hurt you or damages your health. Quite the contrary, if you want to stay healthy, then your body must make use of the autophagy process.

This revolutionary process allows the body to take its damaged and dying cells and recycle them into healthier and younger cells. To put it simply, the autophagy process works similarly to compost. When you are gardening, you get rid of your old useless scraps and molded or rotting produce you are unable to use. But, instead of simply throwing these scraps into the trash, you recycle them into compost to grow new and healthier produce. It is a life cycle that continuously feeds itself so that your garden begins to flourish more day by day, and nothing goes to waste. Your body uses autophagy for the same purpose.

By utilizing the autophagy process, you can help your body to maintain a state of homeostasis, where your cells are consistently being cleaned and repaired. This is especially important in today's day in age when many of us are being assaulted by toxins from every angle. These toxins are in the food we eat, the air we breathe, and the water we drink. Not only are they coming from the outside in, but our own bodies will also produce these toxins when we don't sleep well or make other poor lifestyle choices. Autophagy helps to remove these toxins and reset your body to what it should be.

The main benefits of autophagy include reducing aging and increasing longevity. As the process literally replaces old cells with younger cells, it naturally lessens the rate of aging throughout your entire body and mind. Other benefits include recycling proteins, sorting out and removing toxins that cause neurodegenerative diseases such as Alzheimer's, and increased energy. With all of these benefits, autophagy is currently receiving a lot of attention in the scientific community, as it has a lot of potential in treating some of our most troubling diseases, such as cancer. Many researchers are attempting to find a way to utilize autophagy in the form of a pill to target especially difficult diseases. While this research might still have a long way to go before it is on the market for cancer treatment, in the meantime, you can make use of autophagy in preventing and managing a number of diseases by promoting the process through the Sirt diet. These beneficial effects were well-documented in the 2010 study we previously mentioned.

A study published in 2017 examined why cinnamon is so powerful in improving the insulin response and blood glucose levels, both of which are important for anyone who has diabetes. It is also important for those at a heavier weight, making them predisposed to insulin resistance and high blood sugar. While scientists have long known that cinnamon has a positive effect on this aspect of health, as it has been used for healing ever since ancient times, it has long been a mystery as to why. However, with a new understanding of sirtuins, researchers decided to see if the polyphenol contents within cinnamon were to thank for these powerful healing properties.

The study found that sure enough, cinnamon is full of a number of different types of polyphenols, which are now believed to be the source of positive effects on insulin and blood sugar. What does this mean? Not only can cinnamon help you, but it means that simply by increasing your overall Sirtfood intake, whether with cinnamon or any of the others listed in chapter one, you can improve your health. In order to validate this hypothesis, scientists tested the polyphenol that is found within cinnamon against the polyphenol resveratrol, which is found within grape skin and red wine. Sure enough, scientists found that both types of polyphenols are able to positively affect insulin and blood sugar levels. This confirmed their suspicion that the positive effects of cinnamon are a direct result of consuming polyphenols. However, it is important that I mention that the type of polyphenols found within cinnamon was generally more effective in managing blood sugar and insulin than the polyphenols found within red wine. This is always important to remember, as you can not rely on polyphenols from a single food source to experience the benefits from the Sirt diet, you must eat a balanced Sirt diet with as many sirtuin-rich foods as possible.

The Journal of Nutrition (in 2007) published a study focused specifically on cancer prevention by utilizing plant-based polyphenols. This study focused on the flavonoid class of polyphenol sirtuins. Within the flavonoid class are several subclasses, including:

- Flavones found withing peppers and herbs
- Isoflavones in soy
- Flavanones found in citrus fruits
- Flavanols in tea leaves
- Flavonols found in onions
- Anthocyanidins residing within grapes and berries

All of these subclasses of flavonoids have long been shown to improve overall cardio health and reduce the risk of heart disease, heart attack, stroke, high blood pressure, high cholesterol, and more. Because of these well-known benefits, the researchers of this study were interested in other ways in which flavonoids and polyphenols, in general, may help protect against disease, such as neurodegenerative diseases, rapid aging, and yes, cancer.

In order to examine how these polyphenols work together to fight cancer, the researchers examined how different forms of sirtuin-rich teas affected tumor cells. The results found that certain polyphenols have a synergistic effect when working together, making the effects more powerful than either alone. For instance, green tea and white tea are more effective when combined than when alone. More research is needed to understand all of the different synergistic effects of the various types of polyphenols, but the known results are encouraging. We may not yet know which specific polyphenols synergistically work in cohesion, but we do know that they are more powerful when combined than when alone. This goes to show why the Sirt green juice is so powerful: instead of getting polyphenols from a single source of plant matter, you are combining many different sources of Sirtfoods to get a wide array of polyphenol classes and subclasses.

Not only is it important to consume a variety of the polyphenol classes, but as previously mentioned, it is also important how we consume them. Along with consuming plenty of Sirtfoods raw and without protein, it is also important to understand other factors that may change the integrity of the food. For instance, you may want to drink red grape juice instead of red wine if you don't usually drink alcohol, but keep in mind that you will not experience the same benefits. Sure, you will experience some benefits from the polyphenols, but it will pale in comparison to that of red wine. This is because studies have found that the resveratrol in grape juice is of low bioavailability, meaning it isn't well absorbed or used by the body. On the other hand, the natural chemical process of fermentation increases the bioavailability, meaning the polyphenols in red wine are much easier absorbed and used. Of course, if you are an alcoholic, have liver disease, or unable to drink for any other reason, you should avoid red wine. But, if you choose to drink red wine in moderation, there are many benefits, especially when done in conjunction with the Sirt diet. If you aren't fond of red wine, you might wonder if you can drink white wine instead. Sadly, white wine is much lower in polyphenols, as many of the polyphenols in grapes are found within the pigmentation, such as the peel of the red grape. But, when you have white or green grapes instead, they don't have the same pigmentation, meaning they lack many of the polyphenols that make red wine a healthy part of a balanced diet when enjoyed in moderation.

This study found that the answer to the French Paradox. Confusion on how French people have better heart health than average despite their high consumption of fat may likely be due to the consumption of polyphenols in red wine. As the French regularly consume red wine, which is known to benefit heart health, it may be offsetting their high consumption of butter, which is known to worsen heart health.

Please always be mindful of how much you drink. Yes, red wine is healthy and rich in sirtuins. However, in excess, any alcohol, even red wine, will cause liver damage, weight gain, and more. It is something that most always be enjoyed in moderation. But how much is "in moderation?" This can often be a confusing subject for people, as society has largely begun to accept excessive drinking and alcoholism. A person may be an alcoholic and not even aware, because they believe they are only drinking a "normal" amount.

To put it simply, drinking red wine in moderation means:

- Women drink no more than one 5 ounce glass of 12% ABV wine daily
- Men Drink no more than two 5 ounce glasses of 12% ABV wine daily
- No more than seven drinks total for women a week, or 14 for men.

You may be wondering why men can drink more than women. Is it size? Does this mean if you are a woman as large as an average man, you can drink as much as them? Unfortunately, this is not the case. The truth is that men produce twice the number of enzymes required to metabolize alcohol than women. Due to this, men will metabolize ten ounces of wine in the same way a woman would metabolize only five ounces.

Every now and then, a person might want to let loose and drink more than the moderate recommended serving. If you want to do this, without drinking to excess, it is important to know what the maximum amount of red wine you can drink is. Please, keep in mind that when you "let loose" in this way, it should be infrequent, not something you do on a weekly basis. If you choose to drink your maximum limit, a woman should drink no more than three drinks and a man no more than four drinks of red wine (5-ounce serving) a day. Of course, if you do drink this much in a single day, you should still keep your overall weekly total in the recommended amount.

Hopefully, within the next several years, more in-depth studies on the benefits of the Sirt diet will be completed. Yet, in the meantime, we can see by these numerous studies on sirtuins, polyphenols, and caloric restriction that it is a successful and helpful approach. While researchers long underestimated the power of sirtuins and their effect both on weight and overall health and well being, it can no longer be doubted that they play a key role.

CHAPTER 3: THE POTENTIAL HEALTH AND WEIGHT LOSS BENEFITS

In the previous chapter, we explored the science of sirtuins and polyphenols, and how they work hand-in-hand with caloric restriction to form an effective, healthy, and safe weight loss plan. Not only that, but you also learned that by increasing your dietary intake of polyphenols, you could decrease your risk of cancer! In this chapter, we will be taking the science a bit further to explore some of the most common health-related concerns and how by increasing your consumption of Sirtfoods, you can fight back against them. Of course, I am not promising that the Sirt diet will heal you or that it is a miracle. But, unbiased scientific studies have proven that they are health benefits that can be experienced. Some people may experience these benefits to a higher degree than others; either way, you will find your health benefits from increasing your Sirtfood consumption.

Obesity:

We all know that caloric restriction is one of the classic methods to induce weight loss. Countless studies have proven its effects. Yet, it is also well-known that for some people reducing calorie intake alone is not enough. Likely, this is one of the reasons you are currently reading this book. Thankfully, when calorie reduction is paired with increased polyphenol intake, you can increase weight loss and combat obesity. There's many stories of people losing a lot of weight on the Sirt diet, but Adele's stunning fifty-pound loss is definitely the most well-known success story.

Obesity is currently known as a major threat to the Western world, as it promotes disease, and it can be difficult to combat. Many people try all their lives to reach a healthy weight level, but continue to struggle. This is largely why over thirty percent of the United States population is clinically obese, with the condition affecting women to a larger degree. But, if you, like Adele, are able to shed the pounds with the Sirt diet, not only will it be easier to shop for clothes and experience higher energy levels, you will also be able to reduce your risk of a number of weight-related chronic diseases.

Even if you have not experienced success with

exercise and calorie reduction, you can boost your weight loss by adopting a Sirt diet through increasing your Sirtuin (polyphenol) consumption. Sirtuins have been found to change the way your body's metabolism functions revving it up into high-gear and alter your adipose (fat) storage. A scientific review published in 2010 explained how this process works. When you consume polyphenols, your body processes them the same way as they would your own biological Sirtuins, meaning that they can directly alter and benefit your body's chemistry.

Along with changing how your body stores fat, it will also affect how your cells utilize energy, how the cells burn off fat, how much fat is absorbed, it will promote positive insulin and blood glucose change, and many more positive in-depth biological effects. The review concludes when the scientists' belief that introducing an increased number of polyphenols into the diet is an effective means of losing weight and maintaining a healthy body weight long-term.

Immune Health:

We all know that the immune system is important; you learn about it early on in school. However, most of us never consider our immune health until we get sick, and by then, it is already partly too late. Unless we come down with a cold, the flu, or worse, a disease of some sort, we give little thought to this vital part of the body. But, at this point, all our immune system can do is damage control, trying to fight off the infection so that it doesn't kill us instead. We would be much better off if we instead focused on immune health all of the time so that we can prevent these infections from occurring in the first place. Think about it, would you rather have to try to fight off the flu once you already have it, or avoid ever getting it in the first place? Of course, polyphenols can't take the place of vaccines, antibiotics, and other medicine, but they can greatly help you and strengthen both your immune system's ability to prevent infections and fight off ones you might come down with.

In a 2011 study, scientists administered mice with compromised immune systems with a diet high in polyphenols. For the purpose of this study, researchers specifically used polyphenols originating from soy and green tea, but simply by consuming a balanced and Sirt diet rich in sirtuins, you should be able to experience the same benefits. Through a series of tests, the scientists were able to discover that these polyphenols were able to strengthen the immune system in many different ways. This is important, as the immune system does more than just fight bacteria, it also has to repair cells, prevent and repair oxidative stress, and more. Therefore, these tests showed that the polyphenols resulted in a comprehensive and well-rounded positive change to the immune system, rather than only improving it in a single area of expertise.

Another scientific review examined the effects of polyphenols found within red wine and their effect on the immune system since red wine has long been shown to reduce inflammation, improve heart health, and protect against neurodegenerative diseases. The results were very positive, finding that red wine causes the release of both pro-inflammatory and anti-inflammatory cells. This is important, as while chronic inflammation is damaging and many people experience this condition when their health is less than stellar, inflammation is still a vital part of the immune system. Without inflammation, we would be unable to fight off disease or bacteria. Inflammation, when balanced, keeps us alive. The reason polyphenols can release both pro-inflammatory and anti-inflammatory cells is all for the purpose of keeping the all-important balance of homeostasis. In other words, polyphenols will ensure you have neither too much nor too little inflammation; you will simply have what your body requires.

Heart Health:

Oxidative stress, a leading cause for cellular aging, has been found to be a factor in both high blood pressure and heart diseases. Therefore, scientists in a 2004 study sought to learn if the polyphenols found in tea could help treat overall heart health by repairing and reducing oxidative stress. The results were encouraging, showing that when stroke-prone mice with high blood pressure consume either green or black tea, they are able to greatly lower both systolic and diastolic blood pressure. By the end of the study, the researchers concluded that the regular consumption of tea could protect against high blood pressure in humans.

While the polyphenols in the tea did lower the blood pressure of the mice, if you have low blood pressure instead of high blood pressure, you have nothing to worry about. The polyphenols do not actively lower blood pressure. Instead, they work to maintain homeostasis for your heart health. This means that while they will lower the blood pressure in someone if theirs is too high, if you have low blood pressure, it will not cause it to drop even further.

When a person develops high cholesterol, it causes the arteries to narrow and plaque to build up, increasing a person's risk of heart attack and cardiovascular disease. This process is triggered when a person's LDL cholesterol oxidizes and increases, setting off a chain reaction through the body. Usually, the antioxidants found in plasma prevents this oxidation from occurring, but it is not always enough on its own. When this occurs, a doctor usually recommends exercise and diet to help decrease cholesterol levels, and if the condition continues to worsen, they may put their patient on medication. Yet, while the population of France consumes higher levels of saturated fat (which are known to increase LDL cholesterol) than most countries, a multi-country study revealed that the French still had lower levels of LDL cholesterol.

It was revealed that the reason for this decrease in cholesterol levels was due to the high consumption of red wine frequently enjoyed by the French population. While the alcohol itself was not affecting their heart health, the polyphenols within the red wine were. In fact, it was proven that people could experience inhibited LDL oxidation for up to fourteen days after drinking a glass of wine. The study continued to test other sources of polyphenols, such as cocoa, citrus, and green tea, and found that these too, are able to lessen or prevent the damaging effects of LDL oxidation. When this happens, a person is naturally at much less risk of developing a heart attack or heart disease, especially if they continue to regularly consume a high number of Sirtfoods.

Of course, as always, I recommend drinking in moderation. After all, while red wine has benefits, this is only when you consume the recommended serving. When a person drinks more alcohol than recommended, even red wine, it only increases the risk of all potential causes of death. You will only be shooting yourself in the foot if you drink more than the recommended serving.

Olives and extra virgin olive oil have long been known to have a number of positive health benefits, but this has largely been attributed to the monounsaturated fats found within olives. A study published in 2006 sought to learn if all of the health claims were truly associated with the monounsaturated fat, or if the polyphenols found within extra virgin olive oil were contributing to the positive effects, as well. In order to test this, researchers administered three different types of olive oil to participants with varying levels of polyphenols within the oil. Suffice to say, extra virgin olive oil is the richest in polyphenols, and the more processed and refined a brand of olive oil is, the fewer polyphenols it will contain.

The results were great, proving for once and all that olive oil is more than simply a source of fat, it is also a powerful source of polyphenols. This was proven as all of the participants experienced improved heart health; with the amount of improvement they saw increasing, the more the number of polyphenols increased. To put it simply: those who consumed refined olive oil with few polyphenols only experienced modest improvement. Meanwhile, those who consumed polyphenol-rich extra virgin olive oil experienced a much more dramatic improvement.

Overall, participants experienced lower LDL (bad) cholesterol, increased HDL (good) cholesterol, decreased triglyceride levels, lower oxidative stress, and lower oxidized cholesterol, which causes plaque buildup.

Stroke:
Sometimes referred to as a brain attack, strokes are extremely dangerous. While it deals with blood and many of the same risk factors of heart disease can cause it, it is a separate category than cardiovascular health as

it centers in the brain. What happens when a person has a stroke? A tear in a person's blood vessels or a blood clot results in the supply of blood to the brain is blocked off. There are two types of stroke. These are hemorrhagic and ischemic.

When a person experiences a hemorrhagic stroke, it is the result of a blood ballooning into a pouch of the artery, known as an aneurysm. When this balloon of blood and artery bursts, it causes the surrounding tissue in the brain to be flooded with the excess blood. Hemorrhagic strokes are more deadly, and even when a person does survive, their prognoses are oftentimes worse than those who suffer an ischemic stroke.

The more common type of stroke is ischemic stroke, which accounts for approximately eighty-seven percent of strokes worldwide. When a person develops this type of stroke, a blood vessel leading to the brain is blocked, usually due to a blood clot. As this clot blocks blood flow, it deprives the brain of oxygen, resulting in thirty-two thousand brain cells dying in a single second. Within the span of a minute, the ischemic stroke kills over two million brain cells, and the more these cells die, the worse a person's prognosis will be.

Every year nearly eight-hundred thousand people in the United States suffer a stroke of one type of another, and over one-hundred and forty-thousand of these people die as a result. Women are twenty percent more likely than men to die as a result of a stroke. These statistics are scary, and it is why it is so important to both know the symptoms of stroke and risk factors. Any of the risk factors below can increase your likelihood of developing a stroke, and the longer your list of risk factors, the more your risk compounds. These factors include:

- Diabetes
- Obesity
- High Blood Pressure
- High Cholesterol
- Heart AFIB or Arrhythmia
- Narrowed Arteries
- History of Stroke
- Family History of Stroke
- Over the Age of 65
- Excessive Drinking
- Smoking
- Poor Diet
- Lack of Exercise

The good news is that the Sirt diet can help lessen many of these risk factors. You can lower your weight to reverse obesity, lower high blood pressure, and reduce high LDL cholesterol! A study published in 2017 has confirmed that by increasing polyphenols in your diet, you can also decrease your risk of stroke. This study found that not only do polyphenols decrease the risk of stroke by improving cardiovascular health, they also help protect your brain directly. There is a lot of complicated science that goes into how they help, which we won't get into. But, to put it simply, polyphenols can reduce swelling in the brain, lessen the number of reactive oxygen species (the most harmful type of free radicals) that cause brain cell damage, and more. This means that polyphenols work two-fold to protect against stroke: they both lessen your risk factors, thereby lessening your risk of stroke, and then they also protect your brain cells so that even if you do happen to have a stroke, the severity is likely to be reduced.

Thyroid Health:

While we all frequently hear about the importance of heart, lung, stomach, and other organ health, the thyroid is frequently underappreciated by all but those who have a thyroid disorder. While it may not be a major organ, it is located at the base of the neck that manages the functioning of many of our organs. Your liver, kidneys, heart, brain, and even skin would be unable to function without it properly!

The thyroid is a gland and part of the endocrine system, which produces, stores, and releases hormones for the use of our cells. If it either under produces or overproduces these hormones, it results in a number of severe symptoms that worsen as they continue to get further away from homeostasis. Thyroid hormones manage systems such as:

- Heart Rate
- Breathing
- Body Weight
- Metabolism
- Cholesterol

- Body Temperature
- Muscle Strength
- Menstrual Cycle
- Central Nervous System
- Peripheral Nervous System

The good news is that a 2011 study found that polyphenols are able to improve thyroid function. It can do this in a few ways. This study focused on the effect of polyphenols that allow the thyroid to absorb more of the iodide it requires to produce hormones. However, this does not mean that if your thyroid already overproduces these hormones that it will worsen the problem, as the thyroid does not release all of the hormones it produces. Instead, it waits for the brain to signal it to release the previously produced and stored hormones before releasing them into the bloodstream. Simply put, it allows the thyroid to regain homeostasis.

Type II Diabetes:

While polyphenols have long been underestimated, a study published as early as 2002 did analyze the effects of polyphenols from green tea on individuals with type II diabetes. This is great news, especially since type II diabetes is the most prevalent, and the number of people diagnosed only continues to rise. The results were incredibly successful, finding that these polyphenols are able to increase glucose tolerance and reduce serum glucose levels. Both of these effects were great, but they only improved and increased over time as the rats consumed tea-based polyphenols on a more regular basis.

Another review, this one published in 2015, has noted how a number of studies have shown that a diet rich in polyphenols has time and again proven to be a successful means to combat type II diabetes. This review found that not only can polyphenols prevent this type of diabetes, it can also actively manage and treat the condition in many individuals. Some of the other benefits of polyphenols that help with diabetes include antioxidant and anti-inflammatory effects, protection of the pancreatic cells from glucose toxicity, decreased starch digestion, and more.

Kidney Health:

Many people develop kidney (renal) disorders as they age, which is only worsened due to poor dietary habits, excessive alcohol, and other lifestyle factors. Thankfully, a 2007 scientific review found that polyphenols are able to affect the kidneys from injury, increase antioxidant defenses, and keep the renal cells functioning in a desired state of homeostasis. This was especially helpful in diabetic patients who frequently develop diabetic nephropathy of the kidneys, which was lessened due to the polyphenols. Lastly, the study found that when participants drank red wine, the undesired effects that alcohol frequently has on blood pressure were counterbalanced in thanks to the protective elements of the polyphenols.

Another study examined how the most harmful

type of free radicals, known as reactive oxygen species, is a key factor that causes many types of kidney disease. However, polyphenols are full of antioxidants that are directly able to destroy and counter the damage caused by these free radicals, preventing damage from occurring and helping to heal any that has already been caused. This was found to be especially effective when the polyphenols are consumed through red wine, as a moderate serving of alcohol increases the amount of beneficial antioxidant-based kidney enzymes.

Autoimmune Disorders:

There is a wide range of autoimmune disorders, over a hundred in total, which can all affect the body differently! This naturally means that the way polyphenols help each individual disorder will vary. However, the good news is that polyphenols, in theory, should be able to help every type of autoimmune disorder.

The one aspect that all autoimmune disorders share is that they are affected by the immune system, hence the word "autoimmune." While the purpose of the immune system is to actively protect the body from infection and illness, this is disrupted when a person has an autoimmune disorder. When this happens, the immune system begins to attack a person's own body instead of invading bacteria or disease. By attacking a person's own healthy cells, the immune system damages these cells and causes a wide array of symptoms. But, by optimizing the immune system to attain a state of homeostasis, you can reduce the number of attacks caused by the disorder. Previously, we explained how polyphenols help the immune system to maintain a state of homeostasis. Thus, polyphenols can also help to treat autoimmune disorders.

A number of studies have successfully found polyphenols to treat both autoimmune disorders in general and specific autoimmune disorders. Some of these studies have tested type I diabetes, Sjogren's syndrome, myocarditis, thyroiditis, rheumatoid arthritis, and more!

Bone Health:

It is incredibly important to protect your bone health, especially as you age. People frequently develop osteoporosis at an older age, which results in bone deterioration and bone mass loss. Both of these result in an increased risk of fractures and breaks, which is why many people begin to break more bones when they fall as they age. Not only should the elderly be concerned about this, as some people develop bone disorders at a younger age. People who have taken or have to regularly take prescribed steroids should be especially aware of the risks, as one of the most common adverse effects of steroids is bone deterioration.

Many people think that by drinking more milk, they can increase their bone health, but the truth is that studies have found milk to be much less effective than other methods in raising bone density. For instance, multiple studies have found polyphenols to be especially helpful in increasing bone health overall and both preventing and treating osteoporosis.

Neurodegenerative Disorders:

There are many types of neurodegenerative disorders that can affect people of all ages. However, the most common and worrying for most people is Alzheimer's disease, as we never know if it is a condition our loved ones or we ourselves will develop as we age. It is especially concerning, as Alzheimer's disease is only growing in prevalence each year, with forty-four million people worldwide living with the disease. Thankfully, we don't have to accept that Alzheimer's may simply be inevitable. While we might be unable to prevent it in all cases, studies have shown that by eating a diet rich in polyphenols, we can protect our brain health and greatly reduce our risk of developing this devastating condition.

If you hope to protect yourself from Alzheimer's disease, Parkinson's disease, or a number of other neurodegenerative disorders, there is study after study proving the positive effect polyphenols have in preventing and managing these conditions.

As you can see, there are a great number of conditions that polyphenols can both help treat and prevent, simply by increasing your consumption of them. When you combine dietary increase of polyphenols with calorie restriction and healthy weight, you only increase your health further while decreasing your risk of injury and disease.

CHAPTER 4: EMPOWERING YOURSELF WITH SIRT FOODS

There are many uses and health benefits of Sirtfoods. Whether you are enjoying dark chocolate and wine or tofu and eggplant, you will find that you can enjoy these delicious ingredients in any meal or snack. In this chapter, we will be exploring the many health benefits these ingredients have to offer, along with some practical ways you can include them in your daily life. As you already know, Sirtfoods promote weight loss and weight management, so we will skip over these benefits and look toward other health benefits that they offer.

Buckwheat

Many people do not include buckwheat into their daily diets, but you should. Not only is it a great source of fiber, but it is also high in protein, and the carbohydrates will energize you when your calorie intake is limited. By adding in some buckwheat to your meals, you will help them stick with you longer, keeping you satisfied and energized longer than you otherwise would be. Another great bonus of buckwheat is that it is gluten-free, making it perfect for people with gluten intolerance or Celiac disease.

One cup (U.S. system of measurement) of cooked buckwheat contains more than 5.5 grams of protein, 4.5 grams of fiber, and 33.5 grams of carbohydrates. Along with these larger nutrients, they also contain important minerals such as potassium, magnesium, phosphorus, and calcium. Some vitamins found in buckwheat include vitamin K, B6, folate, niacin, thiamin, and riboflavin. As you already know, buckwheat is also high in antioxidant polyphenols (sirtuins).

Buckwheat has been found to be a grain, or rather a pseudocereal, that is great for heart health. As we all should consider the health of our hearts while we age, we can all benefit from these benefits of buckwheat. Whole grains, such as buckwheat, are commonly recommended to be included in a person's daily diet to reduce heart disease. But, many people only eat refined grains, or if they are gluten-free may eat fewer grains altogether. Buckwheat is a great alternative to other grains, as it is typically eaten as a whole grain, it's rich in deep flavor, and studies have found it to stabilize blood pressure.

The high fiber content can also help in many ways. The fiber helps the gut to digest food more effectively, encouraging nutrient absorption, weight loss, and regularity. Fiber is also important in lowering cholesterol and therefore diseases associated with high cholesterol.

When using buckwheat, you can use either the groats (the hulled grain) or flour. You can make pilaf, pancakes, soba noodles, crackers, porridge, fruit crumble, or even cookies! Check out some great buckwheat recipes later in this book or in my Sirt diet cookbook soon to be released.

Dark Chocolate/Cocoa

A diet that allows chocolate? Yes! However, you can't mindlessly eat any variety or endless amounts of chocolate. While chocolate may be a great sirtfood, it's high in calories, meaning that excessive servings can interfere with weight loss. Thankfully, since the Sirt diet manages calorie control, you shouldn't eat too much if you follow the guidelines laid out in this book. You should also stick with cocoa or dark chocolate 70% or higher. While milk and white chocolate may be delicious, they do not have the same health benefits.

One of the biggest benefits of dark chocolate is the role it plays in heart health. As many of the antioxidant sirtuins found within it are varieties especially helpful for heart health, you will find you can greatly reduce your risk of cardiovascular disease. A study published in 2015 found that when people eat chocolate daily, they have a reduced risk of heart disease and stroke. Another study found that when people eat dark chocolate five or more times a week, they reduce their risk of heart disease by fifty-seven percent.

The consumption of dark chocolate has been found to greatly reduce LDL bad cholesterol, which is responsible for a number of heart diseases. But, not only does the cocoa in dark chocolate reduce this harmful type of cholesterol, the cocoa butter in it has benefits, as well. Studies have shown that cocoa butter can increase HDL good cholesterol. This is great news, as HDL cholesterol is helpful for heart health, as it removes bad cholesterol from the bloodstream.

While it may sound contradictory to say eating sweets can help prevent diabetes, and while that may be contradictory if you were to make such claims about milk or white chocolate, chocolate does have this anti-diabetic effect. This is because the chocolate actually changes the way your body metabolizes glucose. It can also help to reduce your risk of insulin resistance. When both of these effects are combined, it greatly reduces your risk of developing diabetes or can even manage your condition in conjunction with your doctor's treatment.

Do you ever feel happier after eating chocolate? It's not just from enjoying a sweet treat, as studies have proven dark chocolate to have a beneficial effect on mental health! The reason for this is because chocolate activates the neurons in your brain associated with reward and pleasure while decreasing the stress response. Along with boosting your moods, these studies have also found that chocolate can improve cognition and memory.

Of course, you can eat dark chocolate plain or make healthy versions of popular sweets with it, but you can also use it in savory food! Try adding some cocoa to a pot of chili to increase flavor depth, to meat marinades and rubs, into mole that can be used to complement a number of Latino dishes, or even to a sweet-savory salad.

Coffee

You may only think of coffee as a necessity to stay awake, or worse; you might even consider it an unhealthy addiction. However, just like tea has health benefits, so too does coffee. In a single cup of coffee, you can get plenty of vitamins B2, B3, B5, potassium, and manganese.

Not only does coffee cause the breakdown of fat to being a Sirt food, but it can also increase your physical performance allowing your workouts to be more effective. Studies have found that the consumption of coffee leads to a performance increase of twelve percent, so try to drink a strong cup half an hour prior to your workout.

People who drink coffee experience a significantly reduced risk of developing diabetes. Studies have found that depending on a person's coffee consumption; they can reduce their likelihood of developing the disease by twenty-three to sixty-seven percent. With each cup, you drink your risk drops by seven percent. However, you should keep in mind that it's important to stay within recommended daily servings, which is three to five cups. Of course, your doctor will know if you have to alter this daily intake depending on your individual health, so ask them for their input.

Depression is a severe mental illness, which is one of the most common causes of disability in the United States. While it's hard to understand how severe the condition is if you haven't suffered from it yourself, those who have to know just how debilitating it is, Depression makes it hard just to get out of bed each day, just to stay alive. Yet, many people are quietly suffering without ever seeking help. Thankfully, coffee can help. Many people use coffee and chocolate to reduce symptoms, which, in conjunction with prescribed medication, can increase the quality of life. A study by Harvard found that when people drink four or more cups a day, they experienced a twenty percent reduced risk of being depressed. In another study, it was found when people drink four or more cups a day; they are fifty-three percent less likely to commit suicide.

Coffee can be added to sweet or savory dishes, such as meat rubs and marinades, chili, mole and barbecue sauces, roasted root vegetables, red-eye gravy, or even salad vinaigrette.

Medjool Dates

Grown in the tropics, most of the dates you find in Western countries are the dried variety. They are highly sweet and chewy and are sometimes even sold in the form of date sugar to be used in baked goods, coffee, or anything else you might want to sweeten. This is beneficial, as coconut palm sugar has more health benefits than cane sugar. However, keep in mind that it is still a form of sugar and should only be enjoyed in moderation.

A standard three and a half ounce serving of dates contains plenty of fiber, magnesium, potassium, iron, copper, manganese, and vitamin B6.

A large amount of fiber in the fruit is great for your digestive health. It can help to slow down digestion so that you better absorb nutrients from your food while also making you more regular. Another reason fiber is important is because it reduces the likelihood of blood sugar spikes and manages blood glucose levels.

Preliminary studies have found dates to lower inflammation in the brain, which can reduce the risk of Alzheimer's and Parkinson's disease, along with other neurodegenerative disorders. It can also reduce Alzheimer's by reducing plaque that forms in the brain.

Sugar can be added to a number of savory dishes to balance out flavors, and you can add date sugar in these dishes instead. Try adding some date sugar to a bowl of buckwheat porridge, to teriyaki sauce, or even to salads.

Kale

Kale is categorized as a calciferous vegetable, is a member of the cabbage family, and is considered one of the most nutritionally-dense foods on earth. A single cup serving of ale contains large numbers of vitamins K, A, C, and B6, along with the minerals manganese, copper, calcium, magnesium, and potassium. All of this nutrition is packed in only thirty-three calories, making it a great choice to add to your daily diet.

The vitamin C in kale is widely known to strengthen the immune system and ward off illness, but that is not all. For instance, vitamin C is a vital component necessary for the synthesis of collagen in the body. Collagen is an essential aspect of whole-body health, as it makes up our organs, skin, and bones. Kale is one of the best vegetables for vitamin C consumption, and it has even more than an orange. But, know that when heat is applied to vitamin C it is destroyed, so if you want to reap the benefits of this vitamin, enjoy your kale raw.

Vitamin K, while being an important nutrient, is often under-consumed. Thankfully, you can consume all of your needed daily vitamin K, and then some, in a single serving of kale. By doing this, you can ensure your blood clots perfectly and that it is able to utilize the calcium you consume.

Kale is able to reduce cholesterol by containing a substance known as bile acid sequestrants. Naturally, this lowered cholesterol reduces a person's risk of heart attack and cardiovascular diseases. In one study, it was found that when people drink kale juice daily, they lower their bad LDL cholesterol, increase the good HDL cholesterol, and increase overall antioxidant levels. This is just another good reason to drink your green juice daily!

Along with salads and green juice, you can also try making crispy kale chips, savory kale sautes, or add it into pasta, grain dishes, soups, and casseroles.

Rocket Arugula

Arugula is unlike many other forms of lettuce, as it has a much stronger flavor that is distinct and peppery, adding a delicious flavor to a number of dishes. Even if a dish doesn't call for arugula, you can frequently add it in addition to or in lieu of other types of lettuce. Arugula is rich in potassium, calcium, vitamin C, vitamin K, vitamin A, and folate.

The calcium and vitamin K found in arugula are both critical for proper bone health. We are taught the value of calcium all though childhood. But, many people are unaware of the role that is played by vitamin K. Simply put, if you want healthy bones, then you must consume enough vitamin K. Another benefit of this vitamin is that it slows aging in the brain.

The immune system is better empowered when you eat arugula, as the copper in its aid in creating white blood cells. The vitamin C can also reduce inflammation and disease-causing free radicals.

Eye health is important, especially as we age and for those who already have poor vision. In a study, it was found that when carotenoids are eaten in food (such as in arugula) rather than through a supplement that they are able to greatly increase eye health. It does this by reducing the macular degeneration that cause's vision decay.

While many leafy vegetables are high in oxalates, a compound that makes it difficult to absorb the nutrients in the plant, arugula has a very low oxalate level, allowing you to more fully benefit from the high nutrition content.

You don't have to just add arugula to salads and green juice. You can also experiment with adding it to pesto, egg breakfast wraps, pizza, sandwiches, quesadillas, and more.

Capers

Frequently found in Mediterranean dishes, capers are immature flower buds that have been pickled. They have long been used throughout the world in ancient medicine, and now studies have proven that they are indeed great for health.

While more human-based studies need to be completed, studies on animals have found that capers can be used to treat many aspects of type II diabetes. For instance, it has been found to lower blood glucose, blood triglycerides, and LDL bad cholesterol. Simultaneously, it also increases good HDL cholesterol. In these studies, it was also found that capers reduced damage to internal organs caused by diabetes.

Liver disease is a prominent condition that can affect people due to either excessive alcohol consumption or excess fat gained in the liver. Even if a person is thin they may develop non-alcoholic liver disease. If their liver is simply predisposed to gaining weight despite being an overall healthy weight. Thankfully, one study found that when a person consumes forty to fifty grams of capers daily, they can reduce the severity of their liver disease.

There are many dishes that you can enjoy capers in. Pasta, meat, fish, salad, roasted vegetables, there are just a few types of dishes that can be complemented with this flavorful little bud.

Extra Virgin Olive Oil

Olive oil is a notoriously heart-healthy source of fat, as it is largely made up of an incredible monounsaturated, known as oleic acid. This is the same type of fats that avocados are known for. This type of fat has been extensively studied and found to treat everything from skin conditions to cancer. Not only are these all great reasons to make the switch to extra virgin olive oil, but it is also resistant to heat, meaning it is useful in cooking.

Inflammation can worsen nearly every leading disease, whether it is arthritis, heart disease, or type II diabetes. But, one of the benefits of olive oil is best known for is reducing inflammation. One study found that a few tablespoons of extra virgin olive oil are able to reduce inflammation the same amount as one-tenth of an adult dose of ibuprofen. Yet, simultaneously, it is much better for your body than NSAIDs, which can cause organ damage over time.

The second leading cause of death in first world countries is stroke, right behind heart disease. But, a great number of studies have found that olive oil can reduce the risk of both strokes and heart disease.

You can try using olive oil in nearly anything that you would use other oils for. While you should choose extra virgin for its health benefits, know that these health benefits can also impart a slight flavor that you might not want to use in most baked goods. There are Italian recipes for cakes and cookies that specifically desire that flavor.

Parsley

People usually only think of herbs as a source of flavor and not one for vitamins and minerals. But, parsley will surprise you! It is high in vitamins C, K, A, folate, and potassium.

As previously mentioned, vitamin K plays an important role in bone health. You can't just depend on calcium to take care of your bones, as it takes many vitamins and minerals to keep your skeleton strong. The great news is that a single half cup of parsley contains a shocking five-hundred and forty-seven percent of your daily intake requirements.

You can find three different types of carotenoids in parsley, making it a great ingredient to include regularly for healthy eyes.

Test tube studies have found the oils in parsley to be antibacterial. When tested against common bacteria, molds, and yeast, it was able to significantly decrease the damaging components. Another study found that when parsley is used in food, it can decrease the growth of deadly bacteria, such as salmonella and listeria. But, remember, even if you include parsley, you still can't take any risks, always follow kitchen and cooking safety guidelines.

With its fresh flavor, parsley can complement a number of dishes. Try making pesto, sandwiches, salads, pasta, sauces, and more, with this gorgeous herb.

Matcha Green Tea

Green tea and matcha both come from the same type of tea plant. However, the way they are grown and prepared are different, leading to a more intense flavor and health benefits with matcha. When the leaves for matcha are grown, the farmers will cover the plants so that they don't receive direct sunlight for three to four weeks. When this is done, various nutrients in the leaf are increased, thus giving it the characteristic dark hue. The matcha leaves are then prepared differently. While general green tea is brewed and then the leaves are removed, matcha is ground into a fine powder that you stir into your liquid of choice and drink directly. As you are drinking the leaves themselves, and not only their brew, you are able to consume all of the nutrients.

Matcha is able to greatly help liver health, allowing

you to reduce the risk of disease and better remove toxins from your bloodstream. Not only is this helpful for people with liver disease, but it is also good news for the elderly and those with diabetes. After twelve weeks of regular consumption, people experienced a significant decrease in the liver enzyme levels that indicate liver damage in a scientific study.

Matcha, much like coffee, can also improve brain function such as memory, reaction time, attention, and alertness.

There are many ways you can prepare matcha. Of course, the traditional method is delicious, but you might also try adding it into juices and smoothies (such as the green juice), making soy milk green tea lattes, or adding it into baked goods. Matcha is best paired with dark chocolate, so try enjoying a daily cup along with a serving of your favorite 70% bar.

Celery

Celery might be incredibly low in calories, with only ten calories per stalk, but this crispy and fresh vegetables have many benefits aside from reducing your caloric intake. For instance, celery has approximately twenty-five different anti-inflammatory compounds in it, allowing it to greatly reduce inflammation all throughout the body, especially if enjoyed regularly.

The antioxidants and anti-inflammatory compounds can both protect the digestive tract, which will only be further benefited by the high fiber content.

This fiber can slow down digestion to increase nutrient absorption, reduce blood sugar spikes, make you more regular, and remove LDL bad cholesterol. Celery even contains a pectin-based compound that has been proven to reduce stomach ulcers, modulate stomach secretions, and increase the health of the stomach lining.

Try celery not only in green juice and salads, but also braised, like soup, or pan-fried.

Bird's Eye Chilies

A single tablespoon of chilies contains your daily requirements of vitamin C. This is not only great for your overall health and immune system, but it can also improve your hair and skin through its ability to strengthen collagen.

Being low in sodium, high in potassium, and containing folate chilies are also able to reduce high blood pressure. They do this by allowing the vessels for our bloodstream to relax. Similarly, they can affect the blood by preventing anemia thanks to their concentration of iron and copper. Lastly, they are able to affect blood by increasing hemoglobin and thus increasing blood flow. This is great, as proper blood circulation is important for overall health, and it's especially important for people with neurodegenerative diseases.

There are countless ways you can use chilies, both savory and sweet. Try adding them to your dishes more frequently, and you will find that with the time you adjust to eating more spicy food. If you like your food mild start out, adding only a small amount and slowly increasing the spiciness over a period of weeks. Before you know it I'm sure you'll be finding yourself loving the spice.

Lovage

While it might be difficult to find lovage herb in some areas of the Western world, such as the United States, it may be worth growing your own. After all, studies have found that it can help flush the urinary tract, keeping it healthy to avoid problems such as kidney stones.

Lovage has also been used throughout ancient medicine to promote lung help, as it can loosen excess phlegm in the lungs, allowing a person to breathe easier.

And who doesn't want more beautiful skin? Lovage is frequently used to care for skin and treat acne and dermatitis. Adding it to your diet can become a new part of your skincare routine.

Lovage can be used in everything from soup and vinaigrette to ice cream and soda.

Radicchio

Also known as red chicory and red endive, radicchio (like all other sirtfoods) has many health benefits to boast of. This is in part due to the concentration of sirtuins in the food, but also due to other high levels of nutrients. You can get plenty of vitamin K and antioxidants, along with a decent amount of vitamin E, potassium, folate, vitamin C, copper, and fiber.

The nutrients in radicchio have been found to help moderate blood pressure and reduce the risk of heart disease. It can also help reduce the macular degeneration that worsens eyesight and leads to cataracts.

This gorgeous vegetable can be used in salads, roasted, sauteed, or grilled. Radicchio goes great with a large number of dishes and is a tasty side dish.

Soy

For a time, soy was demonized as potentially harmful food. Thankfully, science has shed light on the truth: that soy is a powerful superfood and sirtfood that has many health benefits. It is full of sirtuins, antioxidants, B vitamins, zinc, and iron. Not only is it nutritious, but studies have shown it to have numerous profound health benefits. For instance, multiple studies have shown that the more frequently you consume soy, the less likely you are to develop certain types of cancer, such as breast cancer. The participant's cancer risk was reduced to such a degree that it was shocking, and soy can not be underappreciated.

Soy can also improve cardiovascular health greatly, reducing the risk of heart attack and heart disease while lowering blood pressure and cholesterol levels. This effect is even more profound when you are replacing sources of saturated fats, such as meat and dairy, with soy-based products.

Soy can be used in anything imaginable, both sweet and savory. Let your imagination run wild! If you haven't enjoyed some soy-based products in the past, such as tofu, please don't let that hold you back. There are many other soy-based ingredients to choose from. Plus, many people are unaware of how to imbue tofu with flavor, as is usually done during cooking. Try a new recipe, and you might develop a love for the ingredient.

Turmeric

Turmeric has long been used both for food and medicine. In recent years, science has proven what those in India have long believed: turmeric has powerful health benefits. There are many reasons for these benefits, but one reason is the way it interacts with free radicals. Turmeric contains a powerful antioxidant, curcumin, that is able to fight and neutralize free radicals to protect your cells. But it doesn't stop there. Unlike most sources of antioxidants, curcumin goes a step further by increasing the body's production of antioxidant enzymes. This means that you are able to fight free radicals on multiple fronts for better results.

One of the ways curcumin can benefit your health is by reducing chronic inflammation that leads to many of the world's most devastating diseases, such as heart disease, metabolic syndrome, Alzheimer's disease, and cancer.

You can find many traditional Indian dishes for

poultry and curry that utilize turmeric. But, now that the rest of the world has caught on to the benefits of turmeric, you can find more Western recipes for it, as well. For instance, many teas and tonics utilize turmeric medicinally.

Walnuts

Omega-3 fats, also found in fish such as salmon, is one of the most important fat to consume. If a person doesn't get enough omega-3, it can lead to chronic inflammation and a number of diseases. Thankfully, walnuts are a wonderful source of this important fat.

Walnuts promote healthy gut health, therefore benefiting your overall health as it has been found that your gut health determines a great deal of your well being. Studies have found that a single serving of walnuts daily can increase beneficial gut bacteria.

Whether you enjoy your nuts, sweet or savory, there are a wide variety of dishes to try! One of the most basics you can make is spiced nuts, which can be enjoyed as a snack or top off a salad. Although, you can also prepare a number of other dishes with them as they impart a delicious flavor and a great crunch.

Blueberries

This little berry is low in calories but high in health benefits, such as its effects on the heart and the brain: two of the most vital organs. To help your heart, regular blueberry consumption can decrease LDL cholesterol. A single serving daily over a period of eight weeks was found to decrease LDL cholesterol by a shocking twenty-seven percent in one study. It can also reduce blood pressure by four to six percent over the same period of time. When combined, both of these effects greatly reduce a person's risk of heart disease.

Other studies have shown that blueberries can benefit the areas of the brain that affect intelligence and performance. This can improve memory, among other functions.

Blueberries can be used to make juices and smoothies, to top salads and desserts, or even to make compotes and vinaigrette for savory dishes.

Onion

Onions are another one of many sirtfoods that has a long history of being used in ancient medicine due to its profound health benefits. They have been used to treat a number of maladies such as heart disease, headaches, lung disorders, and mouth sores.

Onions have been found to decrease blood sugar. One study found that within only a few hours of eating raw red onion peoples' blood sugar decreased greatly. Other studies have found that by including onions in your daily diet, you can better control your blood sugar.

Multiple studies have found onions to improve overall bone health and mineral density. One study found that when people consume onions daily, they can experience a five percent, or more, improvement in bone health in a single month.

Onions impart flavor in a number of savory dishes

and are quite versatile, but there are also plenty of dishes that focus only on the onion, making it the star of the show. Onion soup is one shining example.

Strawberries

You can find many vitamins and minerals within strawberries, such as vitamins K and C, potassium, folate, magnesium, and manganese. These, combined with the polyphenols and other plant-based compounds, allow strawberries to boast a range of benefits. They have been found to lower LDL cholesterol, raise good HDL cholesterol, manage blood pressure, improve heart health, increase brain function, improve skin and joint health, and much more.

Strawberries have many more uses than just making sweets. You can also use them to top salads, make sweet and spicy compotes and relish, or top off a dish with some strawberry salsa or mole.

Red Wine

We have discussed thoroughly throughout this book how red wine promotes heart health, but it can benefit other aspects of your well being, as well. For instance, it can increase bone health, increase mental sharpness and response, and boost your gut health.

While there are many recipes that utilize red wine in cooking, keep in mind that this will remove some of the health benefits. Feel free to enjoy using it in the kitchen, but it is not a substitute for drinking red wine.

Black Currant

While grape juice and wine can help decrease plaque buildup, in this area, black currant juice greatly outpaces the alternatives. The high number of nutrients found in black currants can clean out your arteries to prevent life-threatening plaque buildup, lower blood pressure, decrease platelet clumping, and protect the heart's cells against damage.

Multiple studies have also found black currants to benefit eye health by decreasing visual fatigue, increasing blood flow to the eyes, reduce vision loss leading to glaucoma, and increase the eye's ability to view detail in the darkness. A single tablespoon of these berries was able to decrease visual fatigue for a full two hours, as was proven in a scientific study.

Currants can be used to make juice and preserves or compotes and marinades.

Cherries

Cherries are rich and full of antioxidants, sirtuins, vitamins, and minerals, all of which give them an abundance of health benefits. One such benefit is their ability to promote your workout recovery. While both sweet and tart cherries are beneficial, the tart variety is more effective for this. By drinking a little tart cherry juice, you can reduce inflammation, injury, and muscle pain brought about by your workouts. They can increase muscle recovery, allowing you to physically advance with fewer injuries and quicker healing. Some studies have also found that it can increase your exercise performance.

If you suffer from insomnia, the inability to fall or stay asleep, then you will be happy to know cherries can help. They contain compounds that regulate your sleep-wake cycle, allowing you to sleep more deeply and fall asleep quicker. In one study, it was found that drinking one cup of tart cherry juice before bed increased sleep by an hour and a half. Another study found that by drinking tart cherry juice every night, you can further increase the benefits to your sleep.

If you want to experience the workout and sleep benefits of cherries, then stick with tart cherry juice. However, you can still get many other benefits by cooking with cherries. Try eating them plain as dessert, or you can make the compote, roasted cherries, barbecue sauce, and more.

Wheat Bran

Much like wheat germ, wheat bran is packed with nutrients and fiber. In fact, wheat bran is superior to the wheat germ in this sense, as it is lower in calories while containing three times the fiber. It also contains essential B vitamins and manganese. Just adding a couple of tablespoons to your food a day, such as over some soy yogurt or in a smoothie, you can greatly benefit your health.

Wheat bran acts as a prebiotic, supporting your gut health. Studies have found that prebiotics such as this can relieve gastrointestinal disorders such as constipation, bloating and discomfort, hemorrhoids, and digestive tract infections known as diverticulitis. By increasing healthy gut bacteria, you can also boost your immune system.

The most common use of wheat bran is to make bran muffins, but you can also sprinkle it over yogurt, mix it into smoothies, or add it into most baked goods.

Cranberries

This tart little berry has long been known to help urinary health, which is especially helpful as one of the most commonplace types of bacterial infections is the UTI. Some people, especially women, struggle with these painful infections on a regular basis. But, cranberries can help. They contain compounds that prevent dangerous bacteria, such as E. coli, from attaching to the lining of your urinary tract, and therefore preventing urinary tract infections before they can even begin. But, not only can they prevent the infections, but they can also help to treat them after the fact.

Cranberries also prevent infection from bacteria that causes stomach inflammation, ulcers, and cancer. By consuming cranberry juice daily, you can significantly decrease your risk of stomach cancer, among other digestive and urinary tract infections and disorders.

You can do more with cranberries than just make cranberry sauce at Thanksgiving. While it may be best to consume cranberry juice if you strictly want the urinary and digestive tract benefits, you can also use cranberries in cooking. They make delicious marinades and compotes, or can even be added to sweets.

Peanuts

Peanuts are not actually a nut and are referred to as an oilseed due to their large contents of fat. That is primarily made of monounsaturated and polyunsaturated fats in the form of oleic and linoleic acid. This is good news, as oleic acid is the same type of heart-healthy fat that olives and avocados are famous for. The result is that just as these two other foods can help decrease cholesterol, manage blood pressure, reduce blood triglyceride levels, and improve overall heart health, so too can peanuts.

One of the benefits of peanuts is their ability to prevent gallstones. An estimated one-quarter of the United States population experience this painful condition at least once in their lifetime, and many people suffer from them repeatedly. Thankfully, studies have found that peanuts can greatly reduce the risk of gallstones from occurring.

You can make peanut butter, sweet or spicy nuts, or even savory dishes from Thailand and Africa to include more peanuts in your diet. Whatever you make, you are sure to find that it's delicious.

Rose Hips

Often prepared in the form of herbal tea, rose hips are a pseudo-fruit from the rosebush plant. It is floral and delicate, with a slightly sweet aftertaste. A large number of antioxidants and sirtuins in rose hips allow them to help with a wide range of conditions, such as heart health, chronic inflammation, immune system health, type II diabetes, and more.

While rose hips are typically made into tea, which you can purchase as teabags in most grocery stores, some people will even make them into jam.

Dark Plums

Plums and prunes have long been known to have a wealth of health benefits, but frequently people only consider them for digestive health and to reduce constipation. The truth is that they contain many compounds that greatly reduces a person's likelihood of developing a number of chronic illnesses, and they can also help manage said conditions. For instance, they can help manage blood sugar to prevent spikes after eating, despite containing natural fruit sugars. This is due to containing a hormone that controls blood sugar regulation as well as high fiber content. Regular consumption of plums and prunes has been shown to reduce your risk of developing type II diabetes.

Other studies have found that plums can improve bone health and reduce the risk of osteopenia and osteoporosis while preventing bone loss. Not only can they prevent bone loss from occurring, but studies also suggest that they may be able to reverse bone loss that has previously occurred.

It's easy to add more plums to your diet, as you can easily eat a handful of prunes (one-quarter to one-half cup) of prunes daily. But, you can also try making stewed prunes, or breakfast bars full of this sweet fruit. If you don't care for dried prunes, I urge you to try the bars, as they are incredibly delicious.

Red Cabbage

Higher in antioxidants and sirtuins than the more common green cabbage, red or purple cabbage still tastes the same. It is an incredibly versatile and low-calorie vegetable that you can add to a variety of dishes with ease.

Due to its ability to reduce chronic inflammation and lessen lesions in the stomach, red cabbage has many benefits for gut health. It is also high in fiber, which reduces constipation, increases nutrient absorption, lowers cholesterol, decreases hunger, and prevents blood sugar spikes. These benefits combined can prevent many common disorders centered on the digestive tract.

The reduction of chronic inflammation can also help prevent a number of other common diseases not connected with the digestive tract. This lowered inflammation can also reduce pain from a variety of conditions, such as arthritis.

Cabbage is easy to prepare, and it tastes great pickled, grilled, roasted, pan-fried, and steamed. Many cultures, such as Japan, will use cabbage in place of grains when dieting to reduce calories and lose weight.

Eggplant

Also known as aubergine, eggplant has many health benefits from its combination of sirtuins, antioxidants, fiber, vitamins, and minerals. One of the many benefits this can impart is benefits to your heart health. In one study, it was found that both LDL cholesterol and blood triglycerides were reduced with regular consumption of eggplant juice in rabbits. Other studies have shown that eggplant can protect the heart against damage.

In other studies, it was found that eggplant can combat several types of cancer cells. For instance, it may be effective against skin cancer, along with other types.

Eggplants are incredibly versatile, as they can be prepared into dips, gratin, ratatouille, eggplant Parmesan, roasted as a side dish, and more.

Cinnamon

What we know of as cinnamon is actually two different types of cinnamon. Known as "true cinnamon" is ceylon cinnamon, but cassia cinnamon is what most people use today and refer to as cinnamon. While it used to be a precious commodity reserved for royalty, it is now something that nearly everyone can afford to keep in their spice cabinet. This is good news, considering its deep flavor and range of health benefits.

One of the many powerful effects the cinnamon has is to reduce inflammation. This, in turn, reduces pain and the risk of developing a number of common diseases. Another powerful effect it has is in how it relates to insulin. Many people develop a resistance to insulin, especially if they are at a heavier weight. This insulin resistance is a trademark symptom of type II diabetes. But, cinnamon is able to reduce this insulin resistance, allowing the hormone to do what it was meant to do. This naturally reduces a person's risk of developing diabetes, as well as reducing weight retention.

Cinnamon also has a powerful effect on the brain and neurodegenerative diseases. Some of the compounds in cinnamon are able to prevent a buildup of the protein tau that is known for contributing to Alzheimer's disease. Similarly, a study in mice found that cinnamon protected the neurons from damage caused by Parkinson's disease.

While cinnamon might be viewed as a simple spice, its effects are profound. Not only can it be used in sweets, but you can also add it to squash and sweet potatoes, use it in curries, sprinkle it over yogurt and smoothies, or even make delicious marinades and rubs.

As you can see, sirtfoods are rich in nutrients and benefits, and we only went over a few benefits for each ingredient! There are many more benefits that we have not covered here that you can experience. By including sirtfoods into your daily diet, along with other components for a healthy and balanced diet, you can truly experience a range of health and weight loss benefits.

CHAPTER 5: SUCCEEDING WITH PHASE ONE

There are many people who want to jump right into the first phase of the Sirt diet and get to losing weight. Yet, there are many others who may be feeling apprehensive. Maybe you are unsure if the diet is the right fit for you. Perhaps you have a bad history of dieting. Whatever the reason, know that you don't have to jump into the Sirt diet right away. It's not all on the Sirt diet or all junk food. Instead, you can choose to slowly integrate the plan and enjoying more sirtfoods to get your toes wet. This will allow you to slowly adjust, and if you decide to fully take up phase one, later on, you can.

If you slowly get your feet damp by increasing the number of sirtfoods in your diet, and ideally drinking a glass of green juice daily, then you will be essentially practicing the maintenance phase of the plan. While you may or may not lose weight during this part (depending on just how many calories you eat and what else your diet consists of), you can experience health benefits. Look around the world, and you will find that any culture that consumes a large number of sirtuin-rich foods also experience improved health as a society. For instance, many countries across the Mediterranean and Asia have vastly superior health to most people in Western counties. They experience fewer cases of cardiovascular diseases, less cancer, lower rates of Alzheimer's disease, and more.

Along with ideally drinking a glass of green juice daily, look for other ways you can easily add more sirtfoods into your diet. Many people already consume these foods, though they don't prioritize their consumption. For instance, it is easy to add more parsley, berries, olive oil, coffee, buckwheat, and kale into your diet. Try to focus on getting at least a few servings of sirtfoods daily, and you will likely experience the benefits before long.

Another great way to introduce more sirtuins into your diet is by adding matcha tea to your daily routine. If you drink coffee regularly, you can enjoy knowing that the coffee is full of sirtuins and health benefits. But, you can still increase the benefits by adding a variety of sirtuin sources, including green tea. While you could just drink regular green tea that you can buy at the grocery store, as we previously discussed, matcha green tea has many more benefits due to its growing methods and concentration. Try drinking your regular coffee in the morning, and then adding in some matcha later in the day. If you can't find matcha in your grocery store, there is no need to worry, you can find it easily online.

You may be wondering what the cost of the Sirt diet is. The good news is that it is highly customizable. For instance, you can either choose to drink red wine or abstain. If you do choose to drink red wine, then you can decide on which brand to purchase based on your individual budget.

For many ingredients, you can shop around for sales. Most grocery stores offer great weekly sales on produce, so you can look through your local sales to find which stores have sales on sirtfoods at a given time.

If you have a large freezer, you can even stock up on frozen sirtfoods or freeze your own produce if you buy excess when there is a really good deal. For instance, you may see that there's a good deal on cherries one week, so you buy extra and freeze them for later when the sales aren't as good.

Ultimately, the sirtfood diet may be an investment up front, but it doesn't have to cost more in the long run. You can get a lot of sirtfoods at great prices, especially on sale, compared to many junk foods that people usually eat. Not only that, but you can save on healthcare costs, which is especially important if you are chronically ill or live in the United States where healthcare costs are skyrocketing. For instance, in 2007, the average American spent $7,700. This increased to $10,345 by 2016 and is expected to surge even higher to $14,944 by 2023. This is only the cost for average Americans; it is even higher for those who are disabled and chronically ill.

Thankfully, you can make choices in your diet now that will lower your healthcare costs in the future. Many people develop dangerous, potentially life-threatening diseases as they age, such as heart disease, cancer, and type II diabetes. But, if you make a change for the better now, then you can reduce your risk of developing one of these conditions. If you are already chronically ill, then you may be able to improve your condition with the consumption of sirtuins, as they have been found to help treat disease. Of course, the Sirt diet can't take the place of healthcare or a good doctor, but any doctor will agree that what you eat affects your health.

The biggest investment you will have to make for the Sirt diet is in purchasing an electric juicer if you do not already have one. While you may want to skip the green juice if you are looking to save money, I urge you not to. The Sirt diet is not complete without green juice, as it would seriously deprive you of some needed sirtuins, as well as weight loss and health benefit potential. In fact, even if you don't plan to fully adopt the Sirt diet, it is still wise to drink the green juice daily for its benefits, as it can help anyone.

Sure, if you absolutely have to save money, then you might choose to use a blender instead. Although, the texture of the blended green smoothie is not something to be enjoyed or desired. It is a thick sludge, and the texture is so hard to swallow that you can't enjoy the flavor. On the other hand, when you use a juicer it is easy to drink and refreshing, and has a pretty good taste. If you are tight on money, then make a choice for yourself on whether or not you use a blender or a juicer, but it is important to know ahead of time that the difference does greatly alter a person's enjoyment of the drink.

But, if you don't already own a juicer, what should you get? There are three types of electric juicers on the market, each with its own pros and cons. Let's good over each type in turn so that you can make an informed decision.

The most common type of juicers is the centrifugal variety. These are mainly what you will find in your local stores. They work by grating fruits and vegetables into tiny pieces and then using high speeds to extract the juice through a sieve. The fiber of the produce stays in the sieve, while the juice enters a container below.

Centrifugal juicers have the advantage of being widely available on the market, meaning you can find them at different price points and qualities. If you are on a budget, you can likely find a centrifugal juicer that is closer to your price range. These are also easier to clean than the alternative, are quick at producing juice, and don't require you to prep your produce as much due to a large entry point for the greens.

On the other hand, centrifugal juicers don't juice leafy greens as well as the competition. This option is lacking if you want to get every bit of sirtuins and nutrients from the greens. These juicers also tend to leave some of the juice in the pulp, not fully extracting it.

Masticating juicers grind the produce through a screw-like auger, and in the process, sorts the ingredients into two containers: one for juice and one for pulp. These work much better for leafy greens than masticating juicers, and they are better able to extract all the juice from the pulp so that you have little to no waste. As these juicers are of higher quality, they usually have a longer lifespan and longer warranties. Not only that, many types can be used to make other foods, such as fruit sorbet, sauces, baby food, nut butter, and even pasta.

With masticating juicers, you will have to prep your produce more, chopping it up into smaller pieces as they have smaller entry points for food. They also take longer to produce juice and clean. In general, they also cost more than centrifugal juicers.

Lastly, there are triturating juicers. The triturating is at the top of the price range, but hands-down the best option on the market. They operate with a set of gears that grind fruit similar to the masticating juicer, but they work more effectively as they run at a slower speed. This reduced speed means it takes longer to produce juice, but it also means that it preserves the maximum number of nutrients and juice.

As with masticating juicers, you can prepare other foods such as sauces and nut butter with the triturating juicers, giving you the most bang for your buck. But, keep in mind that these will be quite the investment. The triturating juicers also require you to have some upper body strength, as it takes a bit of force to push the produce down into the twisting gears.

Which juicer you choose will depend largely on your budget and how serious you plan to take your juicing. If you plan to continue drinking your green juice daily (as is advised) and have the budget, then it is best to invest in the moderate-range masticating juicer or the high-range triturating juicer. Though, if your finances are tight, then you might have to make do with a centrifugal juicer for the time being. In this case, you usually simply have to buy whatever you can afford. But, if you have a little wiggle room to choose which model and brand of centrifugal juicer that you can afford, then I recommend Oster or Cuisinart. You can usually get one of these for around $100.

At the high range for centrifugal juicers is Breville 800JEXL Juice Fountain Elite, selling at an average of $300. It is highly-rated, made of quality, easy to use, and produces juice quickly.

It costs around the same as the Breville is the

Omega 8005/8006. While the two costs about the same, the Omega is generally superior as it is a masticating juicer rather than a centrifugal. You can use the pros and cons of each juicer type above to decide which you would prefer, but I recommend centrifugal over masticating.

The best juicers on the market are by Tribest Green Star, which is triturating juicers. If you want to get the highest-quality juice with little waste, then this is what you want. But, know that with quality comes a high price tag. They tend to run around $500 to $800.

Traditional Version

The first phase of the Sirt diet traditionally lasts one week. During the first three days on the plan, you cut back greatly on your calorie intake, and consume three servings of green juice daily. This will jump-start your weight loss. The first three days will be the most difficult, but they will be short.

During days four through seven of the first phase, you get to increase your calories to fifteen hundred a day and reduce your daily green juice intake to two glasses.

When planning your meals, it is important to ensure you eat plenty of protein, but this is not a high protein diet. You simply need to keep in mind that just because you are reducing your calorie intake, that you aren't overly limiting your protein intake as well.

Lastly, remember that you don't have to limit yourself to only sirtfoods on the Sirt diet. Sweet potatoes may not be on the list, but you can still eat them, and the same is true for brown rice, avocados, and other foods. While you want to prioritize consuming a large number and variety of sirtfoods, keep in mind that to have a balanced diet, you need variety, and you can't forgo other important and healthy foods. The recipes at the end of this book, and my soon to be released cookbook, are a good example of this needed balance.

Menu:

Day One – Three green juices, peanut broccoli buckwheat bowl, 1 cup of pitted cherries = 957 calories

Day Two: Three green juices, spring salad with strawberry vinaigrette, ½ cup soy yogurt = 946 calories

Day Three: Three green juices, black currant and hoisin roasted tofu with soba, and golden milk = 955 calories

Day Four: Two green juices, West African peanut soup, rainbow salad with lemon vinaigrette = 1,500 calories

Day Five: Two green juices, buckwheat kasha with mushrooms and onions, spring salad with strawberry vinaigrette, plum oat bars, and soy milk matcha latte = 1,474 calories

Day Six: Two green juices, peanut broccoli buckwheat bowls, spring salad with strawberry vinaigrette, and golden milk = 1,410 calories

Day Seven: Two green juices, blueberry nut bran muffins, black currant and hoisin roasted tofu with soba, soy milk latte, and Lindt Excellence 70% dark chocolate = 1,456 calories

My Approach

While the traditional approach is great for people who want to lose a lot of weight quickly, I have customized an alternative approach. With my unique approach, calories are not as limited, meaning you will have less hunger and more energy. This method can be good for anyone who would rather go to a slow and steady pace. Like the traditional approach, my approach has two phases. The second phase mirrors that of the traditional approach, meaning that the difference is solely in phase one.

Instead of only consuming one-thousand calories for the first three days of phase one, you will consume fifteen hundred, including three green juices.

On days four through seven, you will consume two green juices daily and bump your calorie intake up to two-thousand calories.

If you want to try my customized approach, try using the menu I have provided you above, but alter it slightly. Instead of using the menu as I have written, you can add in an extra meal of five-hundred calories each day.

By increasing your calorie count by five hundred, you are able to lose weight at an easier pace, which will be more gentle on your body. Ultimately, only you can decide if the traditional approach or my approach is best for your individual situation. Both the traditional and my approach have their own pros and cons, and only you and your doctor can make that decision for yourself.

85

CHAPTER 6: REACHING YOUR GOALS WITH PHASE TWO

Phase two is much easier going than phase one, as it is meant to help you lose weight more slowly than phase one. There is no set calorie limit, so it is best to follow whatever recommended calorie intake (perhaps with a slight deficit) is recommended for your Body Mass Index or BMI. This may mean that one person eats twenty-two hundred calories daily while another eats twenty-five hundred. If you google "BMI calorie calculator," you should be able to find options to help you find your goal. Usually, these calculators will provide suggestions based on whether you want to gain, maintain, or lose weight.

During phase two, your goal is to drink one glass of green juice daily along with three balanced meals filled with sirtfoods. While phase one lasts one week, phase two lasts two weeks or fourteen days.

Another great way you can increase your sirtuin intake, both during phase one and phase two, is through drinking coffee and matcha tea. During phase two, unlike phase one, you can also enjoy red wine and its many health benefits, although you don't replace your water intake with these drinks. These should be enjoyed alongside at least eight glasses of water daily. This is especially important, as the body loses water when you are losing weight, and you must ensure you replace the water you have lost if you don't want to become dehydrated.

When drinking your coffee, I recommend enjoying it black, as studies have found dairy to reduce the absorption of some of the sirtuins in food. Although, if you dislike black coffee, you can always add a little dairy-free milk or even some date paste or date sugar to make it sweet. Another great aspect of adding dates is that it's an additional source of sirtuins. You can make a delicious and rich coffee creamer with just a few ingredients. The creamer involves:

- Medjool dates – 4
- Cashews, raw - .5 cup
- Water – 1.5 cups, divided
- Sea salt – 1 pinch

1. Soak the raw cashews in one cup of water for at least six hours, or overnight. Pour out the water.

2. Transfer the cashews, remaining water, dates, and sea salt to a blender. Mix on high for one minute,

until the mixture is completely blended with no clumps or pieces remaining.

3.   Place the creamer in the fridge for five to seven days. Alternatively, you can pour it into ice cube trays and store it in a container in the freezer. Simply add a cube to your coffee for ease of use.

While you may simply have to buy whatever coffee you like or can purchase inexpensively, keep in mind that quality matters. To have coffee with the most health benefits, choose organic, freshly roasted, and whole bean coffee, such as those sold at Whole Foods. Try to avoid artificially flavored coffee.

You can choose whatever roast you like, but the medium roast is a good choice as it has more depth and health benefits than a light roast and more caffeine than a dark roast.

Like with coffee, you should avoid adding dairy to your tea to maximize the health benefits and sirtuins. Although just as adding dates to your coffee can increase the sirtuins, by adding lemon juice to your tea, you can do the same. Dates aren't the best choice for green tea, but if you desire a little sweetness, you can add a little genuine maple syrup, local honey, or stevia extract.

As it is generally recommended to only have four to five cups of caffeine-heavy drinks, such as coffee and matcha, I recommend having two cups of coffee in the morning and one or two cups of matcha in the afternoon. Be sure that you don't drink matcha past five in the evening, though. While coffee may release caffeine into your bloodstream quickly, matcha, on the other hand, is slow release. This means that even a few hours after drinking your tea, it will continue to give you a boost. If you drink matcha too late in the evening, it could interfere with your sleep.

It is important to be picky when choosing your matcha tea source. Thankfully, you can find most brands online, giving you a wide variety of options to choose from.

When tea plants are growing, they naturally absorb lead from the soil, which you then consume when you drink the tea. This is important to keep in mind, especially since ninety percent of green tea is grown in China, and much of Chia is effected by extreme industrial pollution.

When purchasing your green tea, choose options that are organic and grown in a pristine clean environment to avoid heavy metals, fluoride, and other toxins.

Kiss Me Organics has a delicious matcha tea that you can buy on Amazon for a moderate price. You can also buy organic matcha from Jade Leaf Matcha on Amazon for a slightly higher price.

Remember, with phase two; you are prioritizing eating a recommended calorie intake with a balanced diet rich in sirtuins. You may lose weight more slowly than in phase one, but phase two is an important time for your body to recover. Phase one offers difficulties and greatly restricts calories; you need phase two in order to recover. Never skip this phase or prolong phase one. After a week of phase one, follow with phase two. If you want to repeat the process, then you can start over at the beginning of phase one only after finishing this phase.

CHAPTER 7: HOW TO CONTINUE MANAGING YOUR WEIGHT AND PROMOTING THE SIRT LIFESTYLE

Managing your weight with the Sirt lifestyle after the first two phases is quite simple. You should generally consume around whatever a number of calories are recommended for your specific gender, weight, height, and activity level. You can learn this calorie recommendation from your doctor or online calorie/BMI calculators. Thankfully, you don't have to try to force yourself to stay within a certain number of calories. While you don't want to overdo this frequently by consuming too many high-calorie foods, as this can result in weight gain, it is natural for some days to be over your calorie count and other days under it. During this phase, you don't have to push yourself to stay within a set range; you can take things easy. Maybe even occasionally, you will allow yourself special treats of your favorite high-calorie or junk foods if it is a special occasion such as a date night or holiday.

During this phase, you should continue to drink one green juice a day, to ensure you are getting enough sirtuins. By this point, it should also be easy to include sirtuin-rich foods in all your meals, as you have learned how to do so through phases one and two.

You will find that exercising will become easier as you lose weight and gain energy, and it will help you maintain weight.

While during the first phase of the diet, you should stick with moderate exercises and focus on not pushing your limits, as your body will be adjusting to the restriction in calories; later on, you can up the difficulty. Of course, you still want to pay attention to your body's needs and follow its signals for when you should rest, but if you want to increase your abilities through exercise, you will have to push your limits to a certain extent. To do this without illness or injury, you should always discuss the matter with your doctor.

While you may choose to train and exercise alone, consider taking some classes at a local gym. By taking these classes or hiring a personal trainer, you can have a workout fit for your individual needs and abilities, and a person guiding you that is skilled in avoiding injury.

Remember to always consume protein after your workout, ideally about an hour afterward. This is important, as the protein will strengthen and repair your muscles, reduce soreness, and boost recovery. There are many ways you can consume this protein, whether with a low-sugar soy protein shake or simply by timing your breakfast or lunch appropriately.

With the Sirt diet, you can lose weight, change your eating habits for the better, become more active, and overall improve your lifestyle. Starting the Sirt diet can be a challenge at first, as all big life changes are, but it is well worth the effort. Listen to your body, be kind to yourself, and enjoy the benefits.

CHAPTER 8: QUESTIONS AND ANSWERS FOR SUCCESS

You have likely found answers to most of your questions about the Sirt diet throughout the pages of this book. However, in this chapter, I will seek to answer any remaining questions you might have so that you can begin your journey to success with ease and confidence.

Can Children Eat Sirtfoods?

There are powerful sirtfoods, most of which are safe for children. Obviously, children should avoid wine, coffee, and other highly caffeinated foods, such as matcha. On the other hand, children can enjoy sirtuin-rich foods such as cabbage, eggplant, blueberries, and dates with their regular balanced diet.

Yet, while children can enjoy most sirtuin-rich

foods, that is not the same as to say that they can practice the Sirt diet. This diet plan is not designed for children, and it does not fit the needs of their growing bodies. Practicing this diet plan could not only negatively affect them physically, but it could damage their mental health for years to come. Anyone can develop an eating disorder, but it is especially true for children. If you want your child to eat well, ensure they eat a wide range of foods, as recommended by their doctor, and you can simply include an abundance of sirtuin-rich foods into what they are already eating. Leave the focus on eating healthfully and not losing weight. Even if your child's doctor does want them to lose weight, you don't need to make the child aware of this fact. You can help guide them along with a healthy lifestyle, teaching them how to eat well and stay active through sports and play, and the weight will come off naturally without placing an unneeded burden on their small shoulders.

For similar reasons, you can include sirtfoods in a balanced diet while pregnant, but you should avoid practicing the Sirt diet when you are pregnant. It doesn't contain the nutrition requirements for either a pregnant woman or a growing baby. Save the diet for after you have delivered a healthy baby, and both you and your child will be healthy and happy.

Can I Exercise During Phase One?

If you use exercise during either phase one or two, you can increase weight loss and health benefits. While you shouldn't work at pushing the limits during phase one, you can continue your normal workout routine and physical activity. It is important to stay within your active comfort zone during this time, as physical exertion more than you are accustomed to will be especially difficult while you are restricting your calories. It will not only wear you out, but it can also make you dizzy, more prone to injury, and physically and mentally exhausted. This is a common symptom whenever a person pushes their limits while restricting calories, but it is something you should avoid.

If you are used to doing yoga and a spin class a few times a week, keep it up! If you are used to running a few miles a day, have at it! Do what you and your body are comfortable with, and as your doctor advises, and you should be fine.

I'm Already Thin. Can I Still Follow The Diet?

Whether or not you can follow the first phase of the Sirt diet will depend just how thin you already are. While a person who is overweight or well within a healthy weight can practice the first phase, nobody who is clinically underweight should. You can know whether or not you are underweight by calculating your Body Mass Index, or BMI. You can find many BMI calculators online, and if yours is at nineteen points or below, you should avoid the first phase. It is always a good idea to ask your doctor both if it is safe for you to lose weight, and if the Sirt diet is safe for your individual condition. While the Sirt diet may generally be safe, for people with certain illnesses, it may not be the case.

While it is understandable to desire to be even more thin, even if you already are thin, pushing yourself past the point of being underweight is incredibly unhealthy, both physically and mentally. This fits into the category of disordered eating and can cause you a lot of harm.

Some of the side effects of pushing your body to extreme weight loss include bone loss and osteoporosis, lowered immune system, fertility problems, and an increased risk of disease. If you want to benefit from the health of the Sirt diet and are underweight, instead consume, however many calories, your doctor recommends, along with plenty of sirtfoods. This will ensure you maintain a healthy weight while also receiving the benefits that sirtuins have to offer.

If you are thin, but still at a BMI of twenty to twenty-five, then you should be safe beginning the Sirt diet, unless otherwise instructed by your doctor.

Can You Eat Meat and Dairy On The Sirtfood Diet?

In many recipes, we choose to use sirtfood sources of protein, such as soy, walnuts, and buckwheat. However, this does not mean that you aren't allowed to enjoy meat on the Sirt diet. Sure, it's easy to enjoy a vegan or vegetarian Sirt diet, but if you love your sources of meat, then you don't have to give them up. Protein is an essential aspect of the Sirt diet to preserve muscle tone, and whether you consume only plant-based proteins or a mixture of plant and animal-based proteins is completely up to you. And, just as you can enjoy meat, you can also enjoy moderate consumption of dairy.

Some meats can actually help you better utilize the sirtfoods you eat. This is because the amino acid leucine is able to enhance the effect of sirtfoods. You can find this amino acid in chicken, beef, pork, fish, eggs, dairy, and tofu.

Can I Drink Red Wine During Phase One?

As your calories will be so limited during the first phase, it is not recommended to drink alcohol during this phase. However, you can enjoy it in moderation during phase two and the maintenance phase.

CHAPTER 9: SIMPLE AND DELICIOUS RECIPES TO GET YOU STARTED

In this chapter, I will be providing you with a number of delicious sirtfood recipes to get you well on your way to success. However, this is only the beginning of the journey. In my following book, The Sirtfood Cookbook, I will provide you with many more recipes to fit any palate.

Green Juice

The green juice is done mostly by weight, as it is more accurate when measuring ingredients such as leafy greens. This means you will need to have a kitchen scale on hand, which can be purchased at most grocery stores for around $10. If you can buy or grow the lovage herb, you can add in five grams for additional polyphenol benefits.

Calories Per Individual Serving: 113
The Number of Servings: 1
Time to Prepare/Cook: 5 minutes

The Ingredients:
Kale – 75 grams
Arugula – 30 grams
Celery – 2 stalks
Parsley – 5 grams
Green apple – half
Matcha tea powder – .5 teaspoon

The Directions:
1.   Push all of the ingredients (except for the matcha and lemon) through an electric juicer. Once the juicer has done its job squeeze the lemon juice into the green juice either by hand or using a hand-powered citrus juicer.

2.   Pour one-quarter of the juice into a glass, add in the matcha tea powder, and whisk until no clumps of tea remain. Stir in the remaining green juice and then drink straight away or store in the fridge for up to twenty-four hours before serving.

Buckwheat Kasha with Mushrooms and Onions

Kasha dishes come in many forms, as it loosely defines a dish cooked with buckwheat or similar soft grains. For this dish, kasha takes a form similar to a vegetable pilaf for a delicious and satisfying meal.

Calories Per Individual Serving: 426
The Number of Servings: 3
Time to Prepare/Cook: 20 minutes

The Ingredients:
Buckwheat, uncooked – 1 cup
Olive oil, extra virgin – 3 tablespoons
Vegetable broth – 2 cups
Red onion, thinly sliced – 1
Black ground pepper – .5 teaspoon
Parsley, chopped – 3 tablespoon
Walnuts, chopped – 3 tablespoons
Peas, frozen – 1 cup
Button mushrooms, sliced – 10 ounces
Sea salt – 1.5 teaspoons

The Directions:
1.   On your stove set a medium-sized saucepan and pour the buckwheat and vegetable broth into it, stirring them together. Add in approximately half of the sea salt and black pepper. Allow the broth to come

to a boil over medium-high heat before reducing the heat to medium-low and covering the pot with a lid. Continue to cook until the buckwheat is tender. It should cook for an estimated ten minutes more. If the buckwheat has any excess liquid pour it off.

2.   Meanwhile, while the buckwheat cooks prepare the vegetables. Add the extra virgin olive oil into a favorite large skillet and saute the onions until tender and slightly golden, about five minutes over medium heat. Put the mushrooms into the hot skillet and continue to heat until the mushrooms are tender and begin to release their juices, about seven minutes. Stir in the peas and remaining seasoning, cooking until the peas are heated through, about three minutes.

3.   Add the cooked buckwheat, parsley, and walnuts to the skillet, tossing it all together. Continue to cook the dish together until the flavors meld, about three additional minutes. Serve while warm.

Peanut Broccoli Buckwheat Bowls

These bowls are incredibly flavorful and satisfying. As it makes four servings you can serve them to the entire family, or store them in bento boxes in the fridge to easily take to work or anywhere else on-the-go.

Calories Per Individual Serving: 541
The Number of Servings: 4
Time to Prepare/Cook: 45 minutes

The Bowl Ingredients:
Buckwheat, uncooked – 1 cup
Frozen peas, thawed – 1 cup
Tofu, extra-firm, pressed to remove excess liquid – 14 ounces
Broccoli florets – 24 ounces
Red onion, diced – 1
Parsley, chopped - .25 cup
Sea salt – 1.5 teaspoon
Garlic, minced – 2 cloves

The Sauce Ingredients:
Tamari sauce – .25 cup
Water – .5 cup
Peanut butter, natural sugar-free – .5 cup
Lime juice – 3 tablespoons
Tahini paste – 1 teaspoon
Sriracha paste – .5 teaspoon
Ginger root, peeled – 1 inch nob

Garlic, minced – 2 cloves

Maple syrup – .5 teaspoon

The Directions:

1.   Pour the water, tamari sauce, and other ingredients for the sauce into a blender and combine it on high speed until completely smooth. Adjust the thickness to your taste, adding more water if desired. Taste and adjust the flavors to your preferences. Place the sauce to the side while you assemble the bowls.

2.   Once you have drained the excess liquid off of the tofu (this is best done with a tofu press) slice the block in half lengthwise, so that you have two rectangular bricks. Slice both bricks of tofu into bite-sized cubes.

3.   Set the sliced cubes of tofu on a baking sheet and toss them with half of the sea salt, baking them in an oven preheated to a temperature of Fahrenheit 400 degrees until crispy, about 25-30 minutes. Halfway through the cooking process flip the cubes over so that they crisp evenly.

4.   Meanwhile, cook the buckwheat. Add the two cups of water into a pan and bring it to a boil before stirring in the remaining sea salt and the buckwheat grains. Cover with a lid, reduce the heat to medium-low, and allow it to cook until the water is absorbed, about fifteen minutes.

5.   While the tofu and buckwheat cooks begin preparing the vegetables. Chop the florets of broccoli into bite-size chunks and then add it into a large bowl

along with the red onion and the prepared peanut sauce. Toss together until the broccoli and onion is coated in the sauce, and then transfer the vegetables

6.   Using a large fork fluff the cooked buckwheat and stir in the minced garlic. Divide the buckwheat between bowls for serving, top with the broccoli mixture, and lastly the tofu cubes. Enjoy while warm.

Spring Salad with Strawberry Vinaigrette

This salad is full of flavor, color, and more than ten different types of sirtfoods. With this salad you can kick your weight loss, and your health, into high gear. It also has over eighteen grams of protein, which will keep you full for hours to come, especially if you serve it along with some cooked whole grains.

Calories Per Individual Serving: 483
The Number of Servings: 2
Time to Prepare/Cook: 7 minutes

The Ingredients:
Kale, curly, chopped – 2 cups
Red cabbage, shredded – 1 cup
Arugula – 1 cup
Carrot, grated – 1
Red onion, finely sliced – .5
Celery, finely chopped – 1 rib
Parsley, chopped – .5 cup
Walnuts, toasted and chopped – .5 cup
Blueberries – .5 cup
Boiled egg, sliced – 1
Blue cheese or feta cheese, crumbled – .25 cup
Chicken breast, cooked, diced – .25 cup
Strawberries, frozen – .25 cup
Black pepper, ground – .25 teaspoon
Extra virgin olive oil – 1 tablespoon
Apple cider vinegar – 1 tablespoon

Medjool dates, pitted – 1

Sea salt – .5 teaspoon

The Directions:

1.   Begin by making the strawberry vinaigrette. To do this add the frozen strawberries, black pepper, olive oil, apple cider vinegar, medjool date, and sea salt all into a blender. Blend on high until the vinaigrette is completely smooth with no clumps. Set aside.

2.   Add the vegetables, blueberries, walnuts, and parsley to a bowl together, and toss them to combine. Drizzle the prepared vinaigrette over the salad and then toss again.

3.   Over the top of your salad sprinkle the boiled egg, cheese, and chicken. Divide out the servings and enjoy immediately. If you wish to prepare your salad ahead of time, hold off on adding the vinaigrette until the last moment to avoid wilting.

Rainbow Salad with Lemon Vinaigrette

This is one of a few salads that can be made in advance, as the vegetables in it are more hardy and able to stand up to the vinaigrette. You will love how this salad is a mixture of fresh greens with roasted sweet potatoes and buckwheat groats.

Calories Per Individual Serving: 793
The Number of Servings: 2
Time to Prepare/Cook: 7 minutes

The Ingredients:

Sweet potatoes, diced – 2 cups

Brussels sprouts, shredded – 2 cups

Red cabbage, shredded – 2 cups

Kale, chopped – 3 cups

Buckwheat groats, cooked – 1 cup

Fresh cherries, pitted and sliced – 1 cup

Extra virgin olive oil – 1 tablespoon

Almonds, sliced – .25 cup

Lemon juice – 2.5 tablespoons

Sea salt – 1 teaspoon, divided

Date paste – 2 teaspoons

Extra virgin olive oil – .33 cup

Black pepper, ground – .25 teaspoon

The Directions:

1.   Allow your oven to heat to Fahrenheit four-hundred and twenty-five degrees while you prepare the sweet potatoes. To do this, add the sweet potatoes

onto a baking sheet and toss them in the single tablespoon of olive oil and half of the sea salt.

2.   Place the sweet potato cubes in the oven and allow them to roast until they are fork-tender and lightly browned, about twenty-five minutes.

3.   Bring the chopped kale to a large salad bowl and massage it with your hands until it is tender. This step makes a big difference, so don't skip it! Add in the cabbage, Brussels sprouts, cherries, almonds, roasted sweet potatoes, and buckwheat groats. Toss them all together.

4.   In another bowl, use a whisk and vigorously combine the remaining olive oil, date paste, black pepper, lemon juice, and the remaining sea salt. Once the vinaigrette has emulsified pour it over your salad and toss until it is evenly coated. Serve immediately or prepare up to one day in advance.

Blueberry Nut Bran Muffins

These muffins are healthier than your standard blueberry muffins, yet more tasty than traditional bran muffins. You will find that the walnuts and blueberries add a wonderful flavor and texture that perfectly compliment the deep flavor of the wheat bran.

Calories Per Individual Serving: 567
The Number of Servings: 4
Time to Prepare/Cook: 25 minutes

The Ingredients:
Wheat bran – 1 cup
Whole wheat flour – 1.5 cups
Sea salt - .5 teaspoon
Baking soda - .25 teaspoon
Baking powder - .25 teaspoon
Cinnamon – 1.5 teaspoons
Eggs – 2
Soy milk, unsweetened - .75 cup
Apple cider vinegar – 1 tablespoon
Apple sauce, unsweetened - .33 cup
Date sugar – .5 cup
Soybean oil - .33 cup
Blueberries, fresh or frozen – 1 cup
Walnuts, chopped - .5 cup

The Directions:
1.   Begin by setting your standard or toaster oven

to Fahrenheit four-hundred degrees. Line a twelve-cup muffin tin and then spray the paper liners with nonstick cooking spray.

2.   Whisk together the eggs, applesauce, date sugar, soybean oil, soy milk, and apple cider vinegar in a large bowl until fully combined. Set it aside.

3.   Stir together the whole wheat flour, wheat bran, cinnamon, sea salt, baking soda, and baking soda in another clean bowl. Once the dry ingredients are combined, fol them into the other prepared ingredients. Gently fold in the blueberries and walnuts, just until combined.

4.   Divide the blueberry nut bran muffin batter between the prepared muffin liners and allow them to cook until fully done and a toothpick once inserted is removed clean, about fifteen to eighteen minutes. Once removed from the oven allow the muffins to cool for five minutes before removing them from the pan.

Plum Oat Bars

These are the perfect way to consume more plums and prunes, and thus get all the health benefits that they have to offer. With a single serving a day you can greatly decrease your risk of many disorders and illnesses. All of these health benefits of plums and prunes are gift-wrapped into a tasty little package that is sweet enough to be a dessert.

Calories Per Individual Serving: 259
The Number of Servings: 9
Time to Prepare/Cook: 25 minutes

The Ingredients:
Rolled oats – 1.5 cups
Baking powder – 1 teaspoon
Almond meal - .5 cup
Cinnamon – 1.5 teaspoon
Soybean oil – 2 tablespoons
Sea salt - .25 teaspoon
Prunes – 2 cups

The Directions:
1.   Begin by preheating the oven to Fahrenheit three-hundred and fifty degrees and preparing the prunes. Add the prunes to a large bowl and pour hot water over them until fully submerged. Allow the prunes to sit in the water for five minutes, until soft.
2.   Remove the prunes from the water and

transfer them to a blender or food processor, reserving the water. Pour in a small amount of the water that you previously reserved from the prunes and blend until the prunes form a thick paste.

3. Add two tablespoons of the prepared prune puree to a medium kitchen bowl along with the oil, sea salt, baking powder, cinnamon, almond flour, and rolled oats. Combine together until the mixture resembles a crumble, slightly like wet sand. You can add more prune puree if it is too dry.

4. Line a square baking dish with kitchen parchment and then press three-quarters of the oat mixture into the bottom to form a crust. Spread the remaining prune puree over the top of the crust, and then sprinkle the remaining oat mixture over the prune puree to add a crumble.

5. Cook the bars in the oven until set and slightly toasted, about fifteen minutes. Remove the plum oat bars from the hot oven and let the pan cool completely. After the bars have reached room temperature slice them into nine bars and enjoy.

West African Peanut Soup

This soup is creamy, comforting, and full of flavor. If you like spicy flavor you can increase the amount of sriracha, using it liberally.

Calories Per Individual Serving: 481
The Number of Servings: 4
Time to Prepare/Cook: 45 minutes

The Ingredients:

Peanut butter, natural smooth or chunky – .75 cup
Tomato paste - .5 cup
Sriracha sauce – 1 teaspoon
Red onion, diced – 1
Ginger, minced – 2 tablespoons
Sea salt – 1 teaspoon
Garlic, minced – 4 cloves
Kale, chopped into 1-inch strips – 2 cups
Roasted peanuts, chopped - .25 cup
Vegetable broth – 6 cups
Buckwheat groats, cooked – 2 cups

The Directions:

1. Into a large stainless steel Dutch oven add in the vegetable broth, bringing it to a boil. Add in the garlic, ginger, onion, and sea salt before covering the pot with a lid and cooking it over medium-low for twenty minutes.

2. Whisk together the tomato paste and peanut

butter in a medium bowl, and then pour in one cup of hot broth, whisking it together. Add in another broth, whisking until combined. Pour the peanut butter mixture into the Dutch oven, along with the sriracha sauce, kale and sea salt.

3.   Allow the soup to simmer over medium-low for fifteen minutes, stirring it frequently. Serve it over the cooked buckwheat and garnish with the roasted peanuts.

Black Currant and Hoisin Roasted Tofu with Soba

If you are wary of tofu, or have been served less then stellar tofu in the past, then I encourage that you try this delicious and flavorful version.

Calories Per Individual Serving: 456
The Number of Servings: 4
Time to Prepare/Cook: 45 minutes

The Ingredients:
Extra-firm tofu – 14 ounces
Black pepper, ground - .25 teaspoon
Garlic powder - .5 teaspoon
Cornstarch – 1 tablespoon
Extra virgin olive oil – 1 tablespoon
Sea salt – 1 teaspoon
Hoisin sauce - .25 cup
Red onion, minced - .25 cup
Garlic, minced – 3 cloves
Cayenne pepper - .125 teaspoon (optional)
Extra virgin olive oil - .5 tablespoon
Black currant jam - .33 cup
Water – 2 tablespoons
Rice vinegar – 2 tablespoons
Green onions, sliced – 1 tablespoon
Soba noodles, dry – 8 ounces

The Directions:

1.   Drain the liquid off of the tofu and slice the brick into two to three slabs, each being three-quarters of an inch to one inch in thickness. Layer the tofu between a couple plates lined in clean kitchen towels and place a couple of heavy cans or pots on top of the upper plate. The pressure will squeeze out excess liquid. Allow the tofu to drain in this manner for thirty minutes. Alternatively, you can purchase and use a tofu press.

2.   Meanwhile, preheat the oven to a temperature of Fahrenheit four-hundred degrees.

3.   Slice the drained tofu into cubes, about three-quarters of an inch in diameter each. Add the cubes into a bowl and drizzle the one tablespoon of oil over them. Gently toss to coat without breaking the tofu.

4.   Sprinkle the black pepper, sea salt, garlic powder, and cornstarch over the tofu and gently toss it until the tofu is evenly coated. Place the cubes of the tofu on a baking sheet and allow it to roast until crispy, about twenty minutes. Use a spatula to turn over the roasting cubed tofu over once halfway through the cooking process.

5.   While the tofu cooks, prepare the sauce. Add the remaining oil to a saucepan and cook the minced onion and garlic until fragrant, about three minutes over medium heat. Add in the water, rice vinegar, hoisin sauce, and jam. Bring the mixture to a simmer over medium heat, and allow it to continue simmering for five minutes.

6.   Begin to cook the soba noodles according to the package's instructions.

7.   Toss the roasted tofu in the hoisin currant sauce and return it to the oven for ten minute minutes. Once done, serve the soba noodles with the tofu over the top while warm.

Golden Milk

This milk is full of powerful spices and soy milk to create a healthy and calming drink. You will especially find this milk helps you to sleep if you enjoy it before bed at night.

Calories Per Individual Serving: 160
The Number of Servings: 2
Time to Prepare/Cook: 5 minutes

The Ingredients:
Soy milk, unsweetened – 3 cups
Black pepper, ground – 1 pinch
Ginger, ground - .25 teaspoon
Turmeric, ground – 1.5 teaspoons
Cinnamon stick, whole – 1
Coconut oil – 1 tablespoon
Date sugar – 2 tablespoons

The Directions:
1.   Stir all of the golden milk ingredients into a small saucepan and whisk to combine it over medium heat. Allow it to warm, while stirring frequently, but don't let it boil. This will take about four minutes.

2.   Turn the heat off and taste the golden milk, adjusting it to your taste. Serve warm.

CONCLUSION

Throughout the pages of this book, you and I have walked hand-in-hand as we examined the science behind the Sirt diet, it's weight loss potential and its amazing health benefits. It's understandable to worry if a new diet being popularized is just a fad with nothing to back it up. But, the truth is that sirtuins and polyphenols have a very real and scientifically-proven effect on human health and weight loss. This has been shown in countless official scientific studies and journals.

You can trust that the Sirt diet works, as many people have experienced a profound change from the plan. While you may have heard about Adele's fifty-pound loss, there are many less famous people around the world who have had similar success. Give phases one and two a try, just once, and you are sure to see results. If you can commit to trying it out for just those few weeks, then you can feel confident in either maintaining the plan through including sirtfoods in your regular diet. You might even repeat phases one and two for increased weight loss.

Thank you for reading this book! I hope that you find the success you are looking for. If you enjoy the delicious recipes in this book, then be sure to keep an eye out for my following Sirtfood cookbook. If you have benefited from this book in any way, please consider leaving a review of it on Amazon.